WHAT A BLIP

A genuinely wise and funny accc cancer and finding meaning on th words what so many women on the cancer feel and never say; this bc ....ce to all who wonder – is it just me? A truly sensitive and inspired story, told with great warmth and generosity of spirit by a gifted writer. **Kauser Ahmed**, PhD clinical psychologist Simms/Mann – UCLA Center for Integrative Oncology

Alicia Garey's *What a Blip* takes you on an honest and at times uncomfortable journey of the challenges one faces with cancer, while giving an in depth, soulful look at not only this disease but the inner fears that arise and the fortitude it takes to stay focused on the result and accept nothing less. Alicia gives direction and tips on how to achieve success, and explores the courage it took to look this massive wild animal in the eye head on without ever backing down.

What a Blip is heart wrenching, endearing, and gives any woman who is facing or diagnosed with cancer extraordinary hope. **Amy Gibson**, Founder and Client CreatedHair.com, Leading Hair Loss Consultant and Wig Designer in the U.S., Alopecia Activist, Talk Show Host, Producer, Author

Alicia Garey's brutally honest look at her battle with breast cancer is equal parts warm and chilling, gritty and poetic, gut-wrenching and funny. From her darkest days to her emergence on the other side, this beautifully powerful writer will sear herself onto your soul and leave you with love, gratitude and above all, hope. **Monica Piper**, comedian, writer, fellow survivor.

What a Blip

A Breast Cancer Journal of Survival
and Finding the Wisdom

What a Blip

A Breast Cancer Journal of Survival
and Finding the Wisdom

Alicia Garey

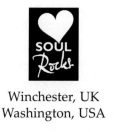

Winchester, UK
Washington, USA

First published by Soul Rocks Books, 2014
Soul Rocks Books is an imprint of John Hunt Publishing Ltd., Laurel House, Station Approach,
Alresford, Hants, SO24 9JH, UK
office1@jhpbooks.net
www.johnhuntpublishing.com
www.soulrocks-books.com

For distributor details and how to order please visit the 'Ordering' section on our website.

Text copyright: Alicia Garey 2014

ISBN: 978 1 78279 225 3

A CIP catalogue record for this book is available from the British Library.

Design: Lee Nash

Printed in the USA by Edwards Brothers Malloy

We operate a distinctive and ethical publishing philosophy in all
areas of our business, from our global network of authors to
production and worldwide distribution.

CONTENTS

~~Becoming Me~~
~~The New Normal Living through Cancer Treatment~~
~~It's Not Over~~
~~Bad Tit~~
What a Blip

Some of the essays in this book have appeared in the following: "Time", "You Cannot Do It Alone", "The Beauty of A Bad Situation", "Don't Be So Negative and Other Interesting Advice", and "Don't Bother Me If You Stub Your Toe" in *The Huffington Post*. "The M Word", "A Beautiful Future" and "The Party" in *Rebelle Society*.

For my miracles Bradley and Rachel,
for Charles, who encouraged me to keep writing and to share,

and for the fighter in us all.

Acknowledgements

To my husband, Charles Freericks, for his never-wavering support, my friend Wendy Hammers for the safe space in her writing workshop and including me in her storytelling line up, my sister Carlie Ramer for her loving encouragement, and John Hunt Publishing for the opportunity. I must also acknowledge the memoirists and humorists whom I so admire; master story-tellers, Jeanette Walls, Mary Karr, and Nora Ephron, and many others who inspired my own expression.

And thank you laptop, for going along for the ride with me, with very little protest.

(No, I'm not going to thank cancer for helping me get a book deal.)

...I hope you will find some way to break the rules and make a little trouble out there. And I also hope that you will choose to make some of that trouble on behalf of women.

Nora Ephron – Wellesley College Commencement Speech

Draft of my letter to the Dyson Guy – James Dyson, inventor of the Dyson Vacuum

Dear Dyson Guy,

Thank you for working so hard and coming up with a series of elegant vacuums that I'm guessing have had a huge influence on the industry. Thank you also for the beautiful fan you invented that has no blades and looks like sculpture. I don't have one but hopefully one day I will.

I think it's time for you to consider taking technology up a notch and applying your engineering skills to help out the female population. Not that vacuums are only used by females but they have probably been your main audience. I don't remember the last time I saw my husband vacuum. Now that I think of it, maybe you could work on a vacuum design that would appeal to the guys too.

But more to the point, I think you are a terrific candidate to develop a mammogram machine that is more comfortable than the current vice grip we ladies have to endure. Cleary you are fond of circles as your vacuums have that pivoting ball and your portable fans are quite sexy and curvaceous. You have a great talent for how the human body relates to an industrial product that requires movement. You could revolutionize this aspect of women's lives and help the medical community, bringing more dignity to what is currently an extremely awkward but necessary and important procedure.

I hope you'll give it some thought.

Sincerely,

Alicia Garey

1

Where I Need Not Worry

I was once only bothered by little things like a cold day or scuffed
  shoes.

I was different then. I didn't know how I would change.

When my fucking hair would come out and poison would fill my
  veins to get better.

I want to escape to a far away land with hills and daisies.

I want to run along in my bare feet

The damp grass staining my toes as I tumble somersaults and
  cartwheels.

I want to skip and hop and fly away into a puff of clouds.

I want to feel the sun on my shoulders and be free.

I want to watch the sun fall below the horizon

Slowly I'll lean back as the first stars begin to peak through an
  endless night.

I want to hear crickets and feel tiny flying bugs around my face.

I want to watch fire flies flicker and glow.

I want every day for there to be time for this place – to run to it
  whenever I need relief from what I know.

Relief from my cry of hope.

As I recover from a horrid thing.

An illness that makes you real. An illness that turns you inside out.

I want nothing to do with it. I'll run and skip away.

I'll go visit the horse stable and feel the force of energy from the
  massive creatures within it.

I'll sit by the pond and watch the ducks float along their glassy
  reflections.

I'll wander to a tree and hug it.

I'll pick up a leaf and notice the browns and golds that fall
  impressed upon it.

I'll be safe on the meadow listening and watching the creatures of
  the world.

I'll be there and never again have to worry.

Never again needing to question a thing.

Strange Guilt

This is a recent Facebook chat with a friend I hadn't spoken to in 30 years. It went like this:

She: Can I ask you a personal question?
Me: Sure.
She: Are you cancer free?
I thought this over for a minute and decided on my response.
Me: I hope so.

The other answer is *today I am*. In the waiting area at my son's orthodontist appointment a little while ago, my thoughts wandered to how I *almost* feel guilty about my successful outcome. That I may appear insensitive to women who have had it worse, or didn't make it; as though I presume I did something right to have not died (there, I said it). All I did was go through the motions and was lucky enough cancer hadn't spread, and that I responded well to treatment. It's damned luck and living in the right decade.

I sat there thinking about this strange guilt, that I shouldn't be tooting my horn because even though many lives have been saved, many have not. I knew I would come back to my computer after the appointment to write down these thoughts. That I feel somehow guilty for celebrating because the fight is not over.

I watched a YouTube video just yesterday about a woman who was diagnosed in her thirties, went through treatment and three months later it had spread. She continues to fight for her life. I don't know what will happen in the future. None of us do.

As these thoughts roll around my brain, sitting there quietly in the comfort of the well-appointed orthodontist's office, I receive a text message from Lisa, my walking buddy (for the

Avon Walk), that she is unable to meet because she is with her friend at chemo and the friend is having a rough time.

It was as though I subconsciously knew not to get too comfortable with my own damned good luck. I'm figuring this woman will in fact get through this. My prayers are with her right now.

And so the story continues.

The drug Herceptin, which was part of my regimen for an entire year is a great example of how passion and funding arrive at success. Had it not been for Dr. Dennis Slamon's development of this drug and the funds he received to continue his work and begin the trials, I would be on a different path. Approved initially for advanced stage (and not so long ago in 2006 for early stage breast cancer) it allows millions of women, including me, the hope that cancer won't come knocking again. The next great development *must* help many more.

Not for one minute am I oblivious to this despite my own good outcome.

The movie "Living Proof" starring Harry Connick, Jr. is based on the book *"Her-2"!* the true story of Dr. Dennis Slamon and his development of Herceptin. As it turns out, my oncologist studied with this great man, and I am honored to have received medical care from the extraordinary team at UCLA.

The thing is, I believe I was treated for a disease in an amazing time in the history of technology and science. From my parents' generation to today, we've gone from treating all cancer similarly until the BRCA gene mutation was discovered in 1995, and Herceptin for the HER2 Positive protein was approved for use in 1998. That is shockingly recent.

I am thankful the medical community has figured out some decent solutions. It can only get better from here.

I believe in science as imperfect as it may be at times. In my case it was a pretty sure thing cancer would have spread. We stopped it. What more could I want? I also acknowledge that doctors are only as good as the tools they have available.

I believe that one day chemotherapy with awful side effects will be a thing of the past. As scientists learn more about those damned mutations better solutions will be available. My oncologist, Dr. Sara Hurvitz, happens to be at the forefront of these studies. One more reason for my gratitude.

Yes, science can help us now with such precision. It raised the expectation I had of myself to be all the more brave. But a life of sanity after breast cancer is nothing short of a miracle. It is true, we've come a long way. It is also true that there is much more work to be done. Until then we'll need to hold on for the ride.

Suspicion

I had put off the mammogram for a while (over a year) since I had been so busy. Went to the appointment thinking nothing of it. Get a call the following week, they need to recheck the left side. While I'm scheduling my hand goes to my left breast. Get off the phone and immediately check. Two lumps. Couldn't believe I had never felt them before, although one is so tiny I could have never known. Face goes white. Heart drops into my stomach. What the fuck?

At the follow-up ultrasound the radiologist looks at me and says she is "very concerned". My face is hot and buzzing and I barely say "But I feel fine". "Good" she says, "You're otherwise healthy which will help you stay strong".

That night tossing and turning, I go through my whole life story in my head. How did I become the person I am today? Despite all obstacles, was I a good person? Had I done enough? How will I be remembered? What can I do before I die? Head spinning, then exhaustion.

Each movement feels like a tragedy. Each thought feels like the last one I might ever have. How would I be strong enough for treatment? How could my body tolerate it? Under five feet and ninety pounds, I can't afford to lose any weight. How would I get through nausea? How would my kids feel about all of this? Would it traumatize them for life? How will my husband move on? How will I say goodbye? Can I work?

Total unpredictability. Nothing is certain. I am at the mercy of an unknown. Seventy to eighty percent of breast lumps are not cancer. Repeat, seventy to eighty percent of breast lumps are *not* cancer. How do women go through this? I somehow thought that because I am thin and eat my veggies and am active and have no immediate history of cancer that I would coast through life fairly well. That it only happens to other women.

It happens to anybody. I am no better and no worse than anyone who is struck by disease. I have begun to question every single thing I do, how I do it, what matters, what doesn't matter. I have a newfound respect for every woman who has had to face this uncertainty and for those who braved treatment, for those who survived, and for those who did not. I could be hit by a car tomorrow. I could be struck by some other illness later in life. I just didn't know I would get this close at this time. I just didn't know.

Even though I believe in taking care of myself I don't like to run to doctors for every last thing. Most ailments are nothing you can't recover from in a week.

This, this is different. This is treacherous. This is powerful. This is bend on your knees please God don't do this to me surrender. This is a total life re-evaluation. This is being at the mercy of the medical profession. This is trusting the help of others. This is real.

Day of the biopsy comes. Feeling oddly at peace with getting it taken care of. The smallest bit of curiosity about the procedure keeps me on track.

Having just started a wonderful new interior design job I should be feeling on top of the world. Then this. This thing that put everything into perspective or took it out of perspective, depending on how you look at it.

I had taken a muscle relaxer after signing the consent forms prior to the procedure, just enough to let me mellow out. Nervous as all hell lying on the table. The technician does her work on the ultrasound swirling the transducer on my skin, over the lumps, watching her screen. I watch too. I see the inside of my poor breast. My small breasts never gave me much trouble. In my teens I was a proud member of the itty-bitty-titty-committee, always took in stride my breasts were appropriately proportioned to my body. Overall wearing lightly padded bras made me feel just right, no complaints. Tender during periods as they're supposed to be.

Now the left one is being taped off readied for poking. The doctor explains every step of the way. First bee sting shot of anesthetic. Not pleasant but not too bad. The doctor positions her biopsy tool, starting to ready for the first one of which I am told there will likely be four. Four fucking specimens. It goes into my breast and comes out with a loud staple gun-like click. I feel a sharp pain as though a knife has been inserted right into my nipple. I yell out and tears begin rolling down my face and I am trembling. The doctors say over and over, "so sorry, so sorry, so sorry". They suspected that one might hurt because of the location in such a sensitive spot. They give me more local anesthesia. They wait for me to breathe, calm down, while one doctor rubs my foot and makes conversation. The three women in the room, the technician and the two doctors are as kind as they could possibly be.

UCLA is a teaching hospital and I learn there is often a young doctor being trained in these rooms. Aside from some whispering about getting the right position of this or that, and yes there you go, they tell me what is going on. I brace myself for the next sample once they have given the second anesthetic a chance to take over. They tell me when it will happen and thank the heavens above it is painless. I feel the jolt of the tool, hear the snap of the "staple gun" sound but feel no pain.

Pain is a bummer. Pain causes any human being to be at their most primal. Pain becomes you. And you ease yourself into it. And you try to pull yourself out. And where the pain is has a psychological effect on how you will respond. That the pain was in my small, delicate breast, that the pain was because we were testing for cancer made it all the more unbearable. But when there was no pain it was serious but not earth shattering. It was taking care of business.

Two more samples to go. Painless and painless. Done. The

remaining necessities of the procedure finish as I continue to keep my hand over my eyes to avoid seeing my breast. Tiny pieces of metal had been placed in each biopsy site to identify for all future mammograms. Little swirls of titanium markers inside my left breast forever and always. Okay, I can live with that.

Then another mammogram to make sure the little metal things are where they should be. Oh great, another squeeze. Good thing I had the muscle relaxer. Feeling a little woozy in a good way and glad for it. Mammogram is done. The biopsy markers are where they should be. I head back to the private changing room and retrieve my clothes from the locker. I take a look in the mirror and it's not bad at all. Small clear bandages over the little holes. A drop of blood. Breast still feels numb. I get dressed and meet Chuck in the lobby where he has been sitting for the past two hours reading a book.

Because it is holiday time, three days before Christmas, if I do not receive the result by Friday I have to wait until the following Wednesday, as the offices are closed. Well if I'm dying it won't matter to know two days later. If I'm not dying it won't matter to *not* know I'm *not* dying two days later. Either way I'm here, I have a beautiful family, a cute poodle, an annoying cat, a new job, a new haircut and I'm alive with an achy breast. Hopefully I'll be alive for many more years. Hopefully I won't die in a car accident. Hopefully I'll live to be ninety-seven like my sweet great grandmother who had her wits about her until the very end, and like her daughter who lived a beautiful life and died peacefully at age ninety-four. If I have a deadly disease I will have to rely on modern medicine to help me live. If only to watch my beautiful children grow into beautiful adults, I have to live. If only to walk out into the sunshine in beautiful Santa Monica, I have to live.

What matters is that up until now I've done my best despite my failings. I might want to consider forgiving myself for the things I wished I hadn't done or the things I wished I'd done better. I have to find that peace and while thinking of myself and all of the overwhelming fear I have roaming through my body there are others who suffer, who need help. There are others who live with pain from tragedy. I have a chance to recover one way or the other. I have that chance. And I will take it.

If I have cancer I will try not to be disgusted with my body. I will try to be kind to myself. It is out of my hands except that the power of good thought and sheer will can make anything happen. I need to believe that this is a blessing. That this is a call for me to re-establish my intent in the world, accept my flaws and possibly try to micromanage a little less. I need to learn how to love myself a little more and accept that not all things are solvable but most things are manageable.

Today is Thursday. I thought I was okay this morning. I took it slow. As the day wears on I feel the anxiety well up inside me. The not knowing, the not wanting to know, the anxiousness of wanting to know is mind boggling. The odds are in my favor.

Silly me, I will feel guilty for having caused my family upset. I don't like to be a bother. I never feel as though I am important enough to allow anyone, including myself, to be overly concerned. If only I could handle it better. If only I were more brave.

I am practicing visualizing the phone call and hearing "the biopsy was negative". I am picturing holding the receiver, heart pounding, and then melting into happiness when I hear the good news. I am afraid of anything else and that my kids might be home when the call comes. That I will see the caller ID and it will say UCLA and I will barely be able to hold still. I want to have enough composure to accept whatever comes.

Right now the world seems to be in a strange holding pattern as the sun shines and the wind blows. I find it hard to focus on much. I find it hard to go about my business. I want to believe the best. I am in between optimism and uncertainty.

Learning the News

The result came so fast. A common form of breast cancer; Invasive Ductal Carcinoma. I *will* get through it. I keep hearing how many women have had it and survived. I was in total and utter shock yesterday. Today, on anxiety medicine resting my body, eating as regularly as I can. Trying to love myself. Trying to accept.

Chuck is a miracle. I know he is scared. But he and I will be a good team together.

Each day is a day I have survived. I force myself to *not* Google, looking for answers. I try to recognize the sunshine, a new day, a good life. Night-time brings fear, darkness, the unknown. I thought I was stronger. From the earliest days of my childhood in New York, and throughout my life, I've persevered despite witnessing my mother's depression and alcohol-fueled rage. I learned to be resourceful, resilient and self-reliant. Now I will rely upon others to help me through.

*You gain strength, courage, and confidence by every experience in
which you really stop to look fear in the face. You are able to say to
yourself, I lived through this horror. I can take the next thing that
comes along.*
Eleanor Roosevelt

By the Way, I Have Cancer

I was diagnosed during my second term as co-president of my
temple, Beth Shir Shalom. It is a small, friendly reform congre-
gation. Our Rabbi had officiated my marriage to Chuck eighteen
years before and our kids had their bar and bat mitzvahs not too
long ago. I became active at the temple volunteering and
ultimately joined the board of directors. I was nominated for co-
president with a fellow board member, which was an honor.
Before joining our temple I had viewed Judaism mostly from the
sidelines. But this wonderful community offers progressive
thinking, beautiful music and our family has been enriched by
our experiences as members.

I felt it right to let the board know before any treatment began.
I also considered not telling them quite yet. First of all I was
uncomfortable discussing my breasts. I mean really, these are *my
breasts*, part of my female anatomy, mostly private, with the
exception of a little bit peaking out now and then. I was never a
cleavage girl. Suddenly I had to talk about my breasts. And not
just talk about them but explain that one was damaged by this
disgusting intruder threatening my life.

But I realized I wasn't going to hide under a rock. This was not
something to be embarrassed about I told myself, as devastating
and personal as it was. At first I imagined disclosing the news at
our upcoming meeting. I pictured sitting before them spelling
out the details with eighteen faces staring at me in disbelief and
realized I couldn't do it. I decided to write an email. That way

they could absorb the shock on their own at their computer, safe from my reality. This also allowed me time to gather my thoughts to consider how I was going to present myself. I didn't want to be the sick person in the room. But if I had to be that person I needed to take charge of how the communication went down. And I didn't want to be in a position of responding to inaccuracies which can, um, spread pretty quickly if people start speculating. This was a new way of expression for me. To reach out, to trust. I went with my instincts and wrote what I wanted them to know and what I needed to hear; that I was gonna get through it.

Dear Board Members,

I have some difficult news to share but I wanted you to hear it from me directly. I will soon have to start treatment for breast cancer. The good news is that it is early. The prognosis is about as good as it can possibly be. I will probably start treatment sooner than later, but the plan is still being worked out. I will be treated at UCLA Medical Center with some of the finest physicians in the country. I'm in good hands. I will receive the benefit of so many medical advances. I am blessed to be the recipient of such a high level of care.

I wanted you all to hear this from me now before anything starts.

So there you have it. I am feeling fine (aside from the heart palpitations and information overload) and have been told I can continue working. That said, I will certainly be looking to de-stress as much as possible.

I have heard such encouraging stories from so many, so that is keeping me going. Your good thoughts will also help.

I am honored to be a part of our special community.
Alicia

Mostly I was already feeling grateful. At the next board meeting I was greeted by kind (and some sad) eyes, and hugs of love and support. It was the first of many tender gestures I would receive from people outside my family.

As I stood around chatting after the meeting receiving those much needed hugs I watched some of the women zip up their jackets or cross their arms empathizing and seeming to protect their own breasts. I was pretty uncomfortable with my new identity as the woman with breast cancer and I did not like being the bearer of such ugly news. I even felt protective of how awful and scary it sounded.

But we've come a long way. Cancer was once hushed. Not that long ago, there were fewer medical options and it was not polite to discuss. I was glad I had reached out because had I not, I would have missed the opportunity to receive their love and I needed all I could get.

I wasn't skipping down the street tapping people on the shoulder to tell them either. My next door neighbor never knew. She is a busy mom with two young girls and I could not bring myself to present the feeling of doom her way. She was surprised by my appearance when I eventually stopped wearing the wig. Even then I wasn't readily sharing. Walking by each other one day her five year old daughter looked at me, then at her mom and said "Mommy why did she cut her hair so short?"

It was time to tell one more person about my breast; one more person who would look down at my chest and then into my eyes with compassion wishing for me to be well.

Why

I'll never know exactly what went wrong. I was *otherwise* healthy and did not have a known genetic link to cancer. There are few cases in my immediate family. Those that did occur were ruled out by a geneticist as having any causal relationship to my breast cancer. I was tested for the BRCA gene mutation and the test came back negative for both BRCA1 and BRCA2.

I'm not overweight; quite the contrary. I've had my share of typical American (junk?) food over the years but overall have eaten well. Not much red meat, lots of salads, fruit and not big on bread although I do enjoy pasta. My diet has been in line with any typical health conscious American woman without denying myself the pleasure of a treat now and then. I don't smoke. I've never worked in a hazardous environment. I was considered to be on the young side at age 46 when diagnosed.

The American Cancer Society writes *"...the causes of most acquired mutations that could lead to breast cancer are still unknown."* I also fell into a subset of HER2 + (Human Epidermal growth factor Receptor 2-positive). The HER2 marker is present in about twenty percent of cases of invasive breast cancer. HER2+ tends to be fast growing and more likely to spread. Great.

Simply put my DNA made an error and my cells did not repair correctly.

Journal of Insanity

The truth is I am terrified. I don't want to look ugly or weak or sick. And I will be those things temporarily. Each day I wake up and remember. The going bald part is completely freaking me out.

This week I will have a conversation with the oncologist and we will talk about the steps I need to take to begin treatment. I will receive a year of intravenous drugs every three weeks, so I will have a port (short for portacath) implanted in my chest so that veins in my arm are not damaged. The whole thing is repulsive.

Last night I was in absolute tears. I cried everything to Chuck. I cried it all out and he listened. I cried and cried and said every single thing I was afraid of. I'm sure it will not be the last time.

I feel like a burden. On the kids. On my family. I feel guilty for the money needed for the purchases to help me through this. The hats, the wig, the drugs.

Clown Hair

I obsess over wigs. I've been searching every website imaginable. Surprisingly there are few pictures of regular women wearing wigs. Only gorgeous models. I had a dream last night that my wig was being fitted and it worked out great. I obsess all day about how it will look. I am terrified that I will look like a clown with a bulky fake head of hair.

Here I am with a life-threatening illness and all I can think about is the wig. The loss of hair is one thing. The wearing of the wig is another. I just want to look normal.

My Other Breast

Another biopsy on the right side. A very small irregularity was seen on the last imaging. This time an MRI guided biopsy.

One must lie perfectly still while images are taken, breast is numbed, specimens are extracted. I cried, there was some blood, but surprisingly I was not as stressed afterward as the first time around. This kind of MRI is awkward. I had always imagined that these are done while lying on one's back, just like in the movies. For breast imaging it's face down with openings on the table where the breasts go and an opening for the face like a massage, which of course makes perfect sense. In my case they had to pad the breast holders because these things are designed as one size fits all. The doctor improvised and piled all kinds of gauze rolls and whatever else they had on hand on either side of my right breast for a nice tight fit. Not to mention I had to hold still and breathe without causing movement, while attempting to hold in my quiet crying as tears dripped onto the face cradle. And of course, I could do nothing about the itch on my nose which always seems to happen when one is placed in such a contraption and told to hold completely still. I was bruised from all that manipulation and plastic machine parts pushing against my breast bone. I'd like to see some improvements on this procedure, please.

Got the call on voicemail, benign. Now my right breast is blue and green, but I'm glad it's done. Tomorrow I go for the echocardiogram to be sure my heart is strong and ready for treatment.

I brush my hair in the morning and mourn the loss I know is to come. I feel the warm shower flood over my head, use up the last of my shampoo knowing I will not need shampoo much longer. I will miss the feeling of my wet hair dripping on my shoulders. I will miss how my wet hair looks sleek, easily wavy in a way it never is when dry. I tuck my hair behind my ears knowing I will not be doing that much longer. Although some women seem to carry off the bald thing with grace and beauty I do not feel I can. I need hair to punctuate my appearance.

Soon very serious drugs will enter my body. Potentially life-threatening drugs, to save my life. But they will work and I will live. Still, I must endure the difficult path toward recovery.

Presented a vision board for a design project the day after the second biopsy and recently consulted on a potential project. I am a rock star. I can do it. I will succeed. I can do whatever it takes. *Still kicking ass.* I feel spirited with possibility.

The Big Question

Every single person asks "are you sure you're going to lose your hair?" *Yes, I am going to fucking lose my hair.* Chuck said he will love me without hair and I will be beautiful no matter what. Even if I don't believe him it is nice for him to say it and nice for me to hear it.

My first treatment is scheduled for next week, the day after Valentine's Day. I can bring a laptop with movies, reading material, a blanket and we can order lunch.

You Mean I Have to Wear That Thing?

Not sure if I can actually go out in public with the wig. It looks fake. It is fake. I didn't go for the expensive one and now I'm regretting it. It is too shiny and top heavy.

What am I going to do? I'm going to have to tell my new client that I have cancer. My head hurts. My brain hurts. I'm angry, I'm devastated. I'm alone. I hate this. I thought I would feel better once I had the wig but I feel like a fool thinking I could fake it. I don't want to be an embarrassment. I don't want to be depressed. I want to have hair. I want to get better.

I want to get through this thing with grace. At least that was my plan. In about two weeks my hair is going to start falling out.

That is my reality.

My oncologist offered two scenarios for treatment. I could have surgery first and then chemo or the other way around because they were recommending chemo either way. Going for the toxic drugs first would enable the doctors to see how the tumors respond and could result in breast conserving surgery, a lumpectomy. I like that idea. Well, "like" is a strong word. I am ready to jump in and do this. I am ready as I'll ever be. Destroy cells first, cut out tissue later. Fine. Let's do it.

Fear makes us feel our humanity.
Benjamin Disraeli

The Day Before First Chemo

My wig will look great. My wig will look great. My wig will look great. My wig will look great. My wig will look great.

I will feel fine during chemo. I will feel fine during chemo. I will feel fine during chemo. I will feel fine during chemo. I will feel fine during chemo. I will feel fine during chemo. I will fine during chemo. I will feel good during chemo. I will feel good during chemo. I will feel good during chemo. I will feel good during chemo.

I will live to be 95. I will live to be 95. I will live to be 95. I will live to be 95. I will live to be 95. I will live to be 95. I will live to be 95. I will live to be 95. I will live to be 95. I will live to be 95.

I will not get cancer again. I will not get cancer again. I will not get cancer again. I will not get cancer again. I will not get cancer again. I will not get cancer again. I will not get cancer again. I will not get cancer again. I will not get cancer again. I will not get cancer again. I will not get cancer again. I will not get cancer again. I will not get cancer again.

I will live. I will be okay. I will feel good. I will live. I will be okay. I will feel good. I will live. I will be okay. I will feel good. I will live. I will be okay. I will feel good. I will live. I will be okay. I will feel good. I will live. I will be okay. I will feel good. I will live. I will be okay. I will feel good. I will live. I will be okay. I will feel good. I will live. I will be okay. I will feel good.

My wig will look great. My wig will look great. My wig will look great. My wig will look great. My wig will look great. My wig will look great. My wig will look great. My wig will look great. My wig will look great. My wig will look great. My wig will look great.

I am going to be fine. I am going to be fine. I am going to be fine. I am going to be fine. I am going to be fine. I am going to be fine. I am going to be fine. I am going to be fine. I am going to be fine. I am going to be fine. I am going to be fine.

I can work and be supported. I can work and be supported. I can work and be supported. I can work and be supported. I can work and be supported. I can work and be supported. I can work and be supported. I can work and be supported. I can work and be supported. I can work and be supported. I will work and do a great job. I will work and do a great job. I will work and do a great job. I will work and do a great job. I will work and do a great job. I will work and do a great job. I will work and do a great job. I will work and do a great job. I will work and do a great job. I will work and do a great job. I will work and do a great job.

The love and support of others is a gift. The love and support of others is a gift. The love and support of others is a gift. The love and support of others is a gift.

My mind will get me through. My mind will get me through. My mind will get me through. My mind will get me through. My mind will get me through. My mind will get me through. My mind will get me through. My mind will get me through. My mind will get me through. My mind will get me through.

I feel love and life. I feel love and life. I feel love and life. I feel love and life. I feel love and life. I feel love and life. I feel love and life. I feel love and life. I feel love and life. I feel love and life. I feel love and life. I feel love and life. I feel love and life. I feel love and life. I feel love and life. I feel love and life. I feel love and life. I feel love and life. I feel love and life. I feel love and life.

Chemo Day

Last night Chuck and I treated ourselves to a low key but lovely Valentine's dinner at one of our favorite Mexican restaurants, walking distance from our house. I avoided anything too spicy so I wouldn't upset my already flip flopping digestive system. What I do know as we sit there eating chicken enchiladas is that we finally have a plan and somehow the unknown of chemotherapy is more bearable than the unknown of the diagnosis itself. That I don't have to wait around for answers and I believe what my doctors have told me; the six sessions of chemotherapy in the span of fifteen weeks will be difficult but that I will get through it and live.

We arrive at the infusion center at 10:00 a.m. It is strangely quiet and peaceful. I had packed a few things I decided would give me some measure of comfort. I love nature so I brought the movie "March of the Penguins" and an adorable picture of our little toy poodle. I have pictures of my kids on my computer so I can look through those to see their beautiful faces. Patients rest on cushy recliners. Family or friends who have come to support them speak in whispers or sit reading a magazine. Chuck brought his laptop and a book.

Two months have passed since I was diagnosed and my first chemo is being given two days before the port surgery so we can get this thing started. This is it. I (still) hate needles. I am seated next to a large wall of windows and look down from the fifth floor and watch children play at the elementary school across the street. First my blood is drawn to get a baseline on my white cells and all of those other numbers I don't understand. Then I am given a series of pre-chemo medications intravenously to prevent nausea and any allergic reactions to the chemotherapy drugs. The first session is the longest they tell me. About five hours. The drugs are dripped very slowly so that if there is any kind of reaction they can attend to it. None of it hurts, in the physical sense anyway.

I wonder how many times the nurses have seen the expression on a patient's face that first time. I doze off from the Benadryl and wake a while later. The thing that keeps me from totally losing it is that this is progress. My battle has begun.

What Rhymes with Constipation

I hate this journal. I hate what it tells and what it has been. I had the port surgery two days after chemotherapy and although many doctors said I'd be fine I wasn't. I was not fine. I was far from fine. The constipation, chills, exhaustion and diarrhea following the treatment for the constipation made me wonder about my very existence. I cannot do this every month. The port surgery put me over the edge. I was terrified. Now I have huge bandages over the areas where the incision was made and the port placed. It feels raw. The anti-nausea and bone pain medicines both wreak havoc on the digestive system. The oncology nurse had given me the mind boggling list of possible reactions and said that only until I go through it would we know how mild or severe my reactions would be.

I feel like a guinea pig prodded, poked, stuffed with medications. And if all of this were not bad enough soon my hair will fall out. I am not sure I can get through it all. I am not sure my life is worth saving if this is how it must go. These thoughts are not welcome but they come. I told Chuck in my moments of deep weakness that I didn't know if I could do it. He just let me say it.

Perhaps God or nature has decided that this is my time. Perhaps that is it. I don't know how strong I am. I don't know how I can go into that next chemo treatment and not have a total anxiety breakdown. I don't want to do it.

Taxotere, Carboplatin and Herceptin

These are the drugs I will receive five more times. Doing my best to eat well so when my appetite goes bad for a while I'll be stable.

On the one hand I'm glad I'm making progress toward ridding my body of this awful intruder. On the other hand I'm disgusted that these drugs are in my body.

Holding On

Saw news footage of a woman in China clutching her small child almost ready to jump off of a bridge. Police came to her rescue and saved the woman and her child. She is crying, clearly distraught and seems to want to continue with her attempt to end her life; in a place of total despair and not wanting to be saved.

Here I am, not wanting to die being saved by medicine. Here I am clutching on to my life distraught over the possibility that I will either not make it through treatment or have cancer again later in life. Here I am losing my hair, saving my life.

My hair has begun to shed. The brush through it this morning brought forth strings and strings of hair. My heart sank into my stomach knowing this is it. My second wig will be ready on Saturday and I am scheduled to cut my hair very short in the afternoon. Each strand of hair represents the eradication of this awful intruder in my body. With each strand I say goodbye to the diseased me and hello to the new me. The cancer-free me. If I look at it like having a cold, or the flu, or a broken arm, it's not as bad. It is a failing of my body that is being fixed.

Losing My Hair Helps Me Think More Clearly

A beautiful sunlit day. Birds chirping. A perfect day. Blue sky, slight breeze. This is why people live in California.

Today I had my hair cut off. The past two days it fell away and only a fine layer remains. My scalp hurts and there was nothing to do but be rid of the hair and move forward. I've had straight shoulder length hair for at least twenty years. Now I have a short cut until the rest falls out. I wasn't ready to shave it off yet.

I am grateful to be alive on this stunning day. I have a beautiful life. My hair will return. It is a small price to pay considering the alternative.

If I die from this disease I'll know I did my best. But the odds are that I will live. This is what I have been told by all of my doctors and anyone who knows anyone who has gone through it. My breast is broken and it will be fixed.

I will treat myself gently, with tender loving care. I will honor myself. I will hold myself to a higher standard of self love. I can allow myself to be nurtured. My purpose is to learn this and continue my belief in being kind to others and that it does wonders in the world.

My New Obsession

Hat hair. Weft. Tabs. Tape. Returns. Scalp. Synthetic. Shine. Spray. Wash. Tangles. $2,000 and up. These are the terms which have been floating in my head. I own a human hair wig. I never imagined making such a purchase. It is very high quality. I cannot wear the wig until all of my hair is gone as I have to tape it to my head to keep it in place.

Hair on My Pillow

Chuck likes that title. My short hair sheds inside my sleep cap, on my pillow, on my shirts, in the shower.

Had chemo number two today. Went well. Came home a little sleepy. Still feel a little woozy. Four more times and I will be done with the most difficult part of the chemotherapy drugs. Then I will continue Herceptin eleven more times which means I will receive intravenous drugs for one whole year. Tomorrow I get the white blood cell shot, Neulasta. Then I will have some bone pain. Hopefully things will go much better for me this round. I know I will feel soreness in my mouth and a sensation that food has sand in it. But last time it was just for two or three days. I wonder if I would have the strength to go to support group tomorrow. Probably shouldn't push myself.

Bones Have Feelings Too

I feel good and I'm nervous the bone pain from the Neulasta shot will set it later and intrude on my happiness. I can't believe this is me but I feel so lucky to be given this chance to learn from this experience. I could not be happier. So much ahead of me but today I am living. And the sun is shining and I am so grateful.

Afraid of the Shower

Already had my hair cut short. Don't know why it was so difficult. I have dreaded taking a full shower knowing my hair would continue to fall out. Bathed in the tub during the week avoiding washing my head. So much hair comes out in the night caps I knew the shower would wash it all away. Finally picked up the human hair wig yesterday. It is as though my scalp knew and this morning released so much hair into my hands. I was afraid to step in the shower and allow the water to roll over my head.

First I let the warm water run over me. My body has become a stranger to me. I am afraid to touch my breasts. I am afraid of feeling anything under my arm pits. I am afraid of the port. But the water feels good. And slowly, gently I lean my head back and allow the water to rush over me.

My hair comes out more than I had anticipated. At first I feel no emotion. I knew it would happen. But then it keeps coming out and I take deep breaths thinking about what I must look like dripping wet at that moment with my scalp becoming more and more visible. I put the tiniest amount of shampoo on my head realizing I don't need much. I barely move it around. More hair falls away. I'm sure to wash it all down the drain not leaving any behind for the rest of the family to see. How awful it would be for my children to see the obvious short pieces of hair near the drain. I push every hair with my toes. Fallen pieces have rested on my shoulders and I'm sure to rinse and go through the motions of wiping it away with my toes over and over until the tub looks clean.

I let the warm water massage my back. I lean forward feeling so strange and outside of anything I've ever known. And then the tears come. They just pour out of me. I'm not sure how I will leave the shower. Chuck has come back home and I want so very much to share my tears with him, to ask for his comfort in this moment. I decide that the steam from the shower will allow me to get out without having to immediately see my face, my head. With my back facing the mirror I put on my towel. I slowly turn and see my face, my balding head looking back at me. I look so small. I am a cancer patient.

I want to run to Chuck. I slowly dry off, cry silently and sit on the edge of the tub. I gather my strength and put on my robe. I decide to wrap a towel on my head like I do with hair. Only I have to do it very loosely and gently since my scalp is still sensitive. My daughter is watching T.V. in our room so I tell her I need to get dressed and she can come back. I close the door and break into tears. Chuck tells me it's alright. He reminds me that this is temporary. That I will get my hair back and I have a beautiful wig. These are true things and it helps dry my tears. The hair seems so trivial and yet so monumental. I haven't even had a lumpectomy yet. How will that go? My God I have so much yet to face. Now I need to get the rest of my pathetic hair shaved off so that I can use the wig tape on my bare scalp. On the one hand I want to be done with this hair loss and on the other I am mourning in slow motion. With each day I see my little neck and my tiny head and I look the way I dreaded I would look, bald and bare and ugly. Once the hair is totally gone and my scalp does not hurt maybe I'll feel better. Today without make-up I'm not looking my best.

An Email Exchange Between Me and My Mother After She Arrived with My Stepdad Unannounced Yesterday:

Dear Mom,

Thanks for the food delivery. It was appreciated.

You need to know that you said something that totally offended me. You looked at my wig and asked me why I needed to wear "that shmata" in the house, and "isn't it hot". Honestly, you need to think before you speak. Do I really need to explain to you that my fucking hair is falling out? Do you think I am going to walk around the house looking like I was in a nuclear disaster? If you don't like my wig I don't care. I would appreciate it if you would keep your thoughts to yourself. If you cannot come over with a sound mind, preferably not drunk, then I would prefer that you do not visit. I know you are devastated by what I am going through. And I know you love me and care about me. Think about that before you decide to say something so ridiculous. And if you think I'm overreacting, too bad. I'm not.

In the future, I hope you can figure out how to be more sensitive. Thanks.

Alicia

I guess I was a little upset.

My Mother's Response:

Alicia, I'm sorry if I offended you. I do realize what you are going through and that you are super sensitive. I'm glad on the other hand that you can finally express your feelings directly to me. I understand that your hair is falling out and that it's driving you crazy; however as your mother I am entitled to think that you have a beautiful face. I don't know what I would do if I were in your situation, therefore, I don't know how I would react. I apologize profusely for having offended you. That's the last thing I want to do. I can only hope you accept my apology. I truly want and wish the best for you.

Much love, Mom.

"*Hair falling out and driving me crazy*" was an understatement. Apology for comment, accepted.

Thank You

To the woman who cut her hair off so I could have it. So that I can get up tomorrow morning and put make-up on and put hair on my patchy baldness. So that I can have a sense of self. Thank you for being selfless, for giving of your beautiful shiny, silky locks. Thank you whoever you are, wherever you are. You have given of yourself in such a precious way. Such a personal way. I wish I could hug you. Instead I will take care of the golden thread falsely attached to me at this moment.

Four More Times

Four more times I must endure the feeling of aches in my bones, constipation and diarrhea, dizziness, ringing in the ears, tongue soreness, sleepiness. And for those things not including of course hair loss and possible eyebrow thinning I get my life back in exchange.

This is a strange land. I can't even think of the possibility that even five years ago Herceptin was still being studied. This is the incredible thing. This is a story to tell. This is a miracle. Or living in the right decade at the right time. As much as I hate this journal I must put my thoughts down and record this time in my life.

Maybe one day I will connect the dots as an expression of strength and forgiveness. To forgive my body for doing this to me. To be grateful that I will see my children grow. To look forward to going on a cruise. To hopefully one day go to Japan.

Tomorrow morning I'm getting my remaining hair shaved off. It is a pitiful sight these days. Nothing left in the front center, balding on the sides. Very ugly. And makes it hard to manage the wig tape.

To Blend in or Not to Blend in, That is the Question

Went to temple last night. Saw my reflection with my wig and became extremely self-conscious. A few people were there who know my situation. One woman looked at me, asked how I was doing and commented that I look good. As if to say *I see your fake hair and you look okay.* Or was she saying *you look better than I thought for someone with cancer.* Or was she saying *you look terrible and so I will compliment you so you feel better.* (Note to self: learn to accept a compliment.) She had never, ever, before commented on how I look. The awkwardness was painful. And it also feels like a charade. On the one hand I want to blend in. On the other hand for those who do know I want to scream out, *yes, I am going through this and guess what, this is fake hair and I'm still here and I feel alive and beautiful and blessed.*

Progress

Nothing in life is to be feared, it is only to be understood.
Now is the time to understand more, so that we may fear less.
Marie Curie

Who Am I to Not Get Cancer?

I was simply going about my business and the reality of life caught up with me. It's a hard lesson.

I will have to learn to live in the moment. I am here today. I am here and doing my best.

I am afraid but I am also in awe. In awe of the doctors, of how my body can continue and how I am able to get up each day and do this.

I give myself permission to cry, to feel, to be angry, to want, to express.

Empowered by Letting Go

Feeling good these days. Feeling normal. I find that I keep having to tell people that I'm actually okay. That I'm not hiding under a rock. That I am functioning. It is sometimes awkward for people. But my treatment has been pretty darn good so far despite the emotional roller coaster. Of course I have so much more to go. Surgery, more medications, more exams, MRIs. But I do feel less resistant and more empowered by letting go. Isn't that strange. *Empowered by letting go.* That is a good title. I like it.

What I do know is that my tumors are responding and after a year of crap I will live.

This experience has better prepared me for the prospect of dying. It allows me to live now and accept that in fact one day I will die. Empowered By Letting Go. Funny.

Stuff I Want to Do or Want Someone to Do
Go to the Phillip Johnson Glass House in Connecticut
Visit Camp Pointelle in Pennsylvania (some of the happiest days
    of my childhood)
Write something about the C experience
Have living room and hallway painted
Go to Japan
Exercise regularly
Have a house somewhere near a lake and total quiet
Have my home cleaned by a service every week

Also
Buy a poodle pin (in honor of our adorable poodle)

Halfway
Recovering from treatment number three. Yesterday slept almost
all day. Today I took a bath, put on make-up, found clothes that
hide the port, put on my wig and here I sit. Should probably take
Xanax. Wish I didn't have cancer. Can't believe I have cancer.
Can't believe I am going through this. And yet the sun is shining
and I am here. I go through periods of extreme sadness. Then I
feel lucky to be alive.

Worked on my website this past week. Good to do but strange
to think about my future. To do something that benefits my
future with all of the unknowns I now face. After all of these
disgusting drugs I have surgery.

I sweat every night. I wake up with sweat in between my fingers.

How

I read somewhere that holding in anger and resentment can set the stage for cancer cells. I think this has something to do with stress and cortisol which is a stress hormone and if elevated for extended periods of time can be detrimental. Perhaps this is what happened to me. How do I let it go? How do I heal? On the one hand I believe in scientific proof that cancer happens to anyone as we are living organisms. On the other hand I believe there is a connection of mind and body and how we hold ourselves in the world affects the health of the body. It is easy to get caught up in negative thinking.

I do feel that this whole experience is an opportunity to be open to change. I guess that is because I have been forced to change. As many people have acknowledged, in the oddest way, it is a gift. Eventually I will untangle myself from this part of my life and move on. But each experience, whether good or bad, painful or happy is a chance to learn and grow.

Is This Just a Bad Dream?

Woke up this morning and forgot I didn't have hair. Thank God for my gorgeous wig. The hygienist at the dentist yesterday was shocked when I told her it was a wig after she complimented me on my hair cut. Pretty cool. Makes me feel a little better about that part of the situation.

Where Have I Gone?

Mishap with my website. Now no project pictures exist. It is as though I do not exist. All of my work erased. Of course I have the photos but it is sad. Like I am partially non-existent which is exactly how I feel. Like I am half me. It isn't easy these days with all that I am going through. But each day comes.

Each day is my opportunity to get off my ass and do something.

Two More

Today is the day after treatment. I have two more left. I received the Neulasta shot and took my final dose of the steroid Decadron for this round. The steroid makes me hyper for a day or two and then I get bloated from water retention. I took my Claritin (oddly enough it relieves bone pain) and washed my wig.

I am moving forward. I am bald. But I am alive. My project is moving forward and I made changes to my website. I crafted a newsletter which will come out tomorrow morning. I am living. My website was down and I was feeling half whole. But things are working again and I feel I am part of the earth. More and more I am able to accept what is happening to me. I hear great stories of success with this thing and I become inspired, hopeful. I become sad sometimes too. Sad that this happened, and how it scared the kids. And how it has slowed me down. But I must accept all that has come with this and know that I will be even stronger. I never imagined I could be stronger. I thought I had worked out so much. And now I have this.

My Teenagers

I never walk around bald because my kids do not want to see me that way. I spare them.

It is not lost on me that as I brave this part of my life my two teenagers have their whole lives ahead of them. Everything is a possibility. I do not want them to feel defeated by this thing I have to go through. So I forge ahead for them. I will create the most normal environment possible in a time that feels anything but normal. All that I do, I do so they can move forward. When my hair grows again perhaps they'll accept me again. I feel their distance. I'm sure it is fear. I feel it. I understand it. How terrifying it must be. I see in them all of the possibility that I saw in my young life. I have a hard time lately seeing my own future. I have a hard time believing that I will live after this phase in a way that is truly living. I want for them every spec of goodness there can be. My bald head and sick body cannot stand in their way.

Jealous (and tired)

I'm jealous of everyone living their lives. I miss being normal. I look like an alien. I hide my feelings so my family does not have to feel my pain. I don't want to drag them down with me. I am tired of this. I question if I am worth saving. And that is sad. The truth is, in the end, only I can find my own self-worth. No one can do it for me. I feel sorry for myself. I guess I deserve that.

It is not only the physical aftermath of chemo. It is the separation from my normal life. It is the doctor appointments, the unknown surgery ahead. It is anticipating the five years of Tamoxifen. It is the hot flashes, the baldness, the digestive issues. It is carefully selecting clothing each day that hides the port. It is putting on the appearance of being normal while I am actually so afraid.

Want to go away to an island somewhere. Really hard to hold my head up high these days. People think I'm strong. I'm not. I'm weak and tired and angry and sad. I'm totally withdrawn and moody. I'm barely surviving. I am so tired of pretending to be strong.

Yesterday was Not So Good

Had a more normal day today. When I am feeling physically at my worst it's rough. Today feeling much better. Tomorrow is my follow-up with oncology.

I have a list of ailments to report:

eye twitching
legs get swollen
hot flashes and night sweats
cold feet
numb toe
slightly numb fingertips
thigh aches

It's all "normal" and expected from treatment so I won't worry. Oh, and heart palpitations.

The Big Fake Out

I have become as ugly as I've ever been and I still have to accept myself.

To the outside world I present a decent picture. This casts the somewhat inaccurate perception that all is well. Each and every day I deal with small, strange effects of chemotherapy. I brave the open sea of stepping outside that front door. I talk myself into facing the sunshine, talking to people as though I am fine.

I must learn to keep my eye on the big picture and yet be okay with each small moment. Be okay right now with my swollen eye from a sty, blotchy skin, fake hair, swollen feet, ringing ears. This is me right now. And I can have a beautiful day. I have my legs, my arms, my eyes, my brain.

A Typical Thursday

Went to support group today. Good to get thoughts out that swim around in my head. Always good to find out my struggles are practically universal. I am trying not to panic about surgery. About radiation affecting my heart. About keeping up my spirits for the kids. About not spending too much money. About having zero interest in sex.

I am so terrified of the next steps in this awful journey. I have my second to last chemo next week. Then more tests to see the progress. Then surgical consult. Then surgery decisions. What if my breast cannot be saved? Will I wind up having a double mastectomy? So many decisions. So much fear.

On the one hand it would seem I should be so grateful to be alive and have a chance to continue. To see my children grow. On the other hand this is so hard, so devastating, I can't bear it. I can't stand to know that my body is being tortured.

Chuck is the most patient person I know. We go about our daily responsibilities raising two kids. It is a challenge. They are great kids but are going through so much just by being teenagers. What a difficult time to see their mom go through this.

My stupid little breasts. I hate them.

Happy Tastebuds

Sometimes I think, fuck it. I ate badly today. I feel like well, I've made it this far and I want to enjoy that sugar, that salt, bread, pasta, wine, candy, chocolate, doughnut, whatever. Not that I like to overeat. But food has become one of life's few pleasures. I can't escape the dread I feel having to go to my next chemo session. I get extremely anxious days before.

One More Ass-Kicking

Treatment number five done. One more to go.

What a Girl Wants

Mother's Day weekend. Just ordered food in. Had a craving for shrimp scampi but ordered fettuccini alfredo as there was no scampi on the menu.

So, so tired of this cancer thing. So tired of feeling sorry for myself. So tired of feeling achy and swelled up and foul taste in mouth. So tired of being in survivor mode.

Today the weather was beautiful. A lovely day. It will be a lovely weekend. No matter what.

Last One

Well, I still have to go back for the Herceptin eleven more times but tomorrow will be the last full chemo. I have to recover one...more...time.

The Day We've Been Waiting For

MRI complete. Moving forward. Feeling okay. Ringing in ears, a little tired and achy. Hopefully good news will come from MRI and we'll know our next steps. I will get through this. I will be better. My hair will grow, my eyelashes will grow. I will feel strong again. I will feel like me again and maybe even *better*.

Day Ten after Last Round

Usual side effects like clockwork; edema, rash on face. The great news is that the tumors are gone. No suspicious tissue found in the MRI. I burst into tears when the nurse told me the news and gave me the printed report. I still have fear that it could come back. How can I live with that? I guess the farther away I am from danger the better I will feel.

All of the Good Things

All throughout this time of illness, fear, shock, sadness, strength, recovery and determination, many wonderful things have happened. Although I live in daily fear and sadness under the surface my son celebrated with his confirmation class at the temple, my daughter graduated middle school, my sister is due to have her first child in October and life in general is a gift. I had a scare of a blood clot in my leg, but thankfully all is well. I must look forward with courage as I head toward the lumpectomy which is scheduled for early July. I am terrified but with chemo behind me I should be glad. One or two people said that I would look back on all of this and it would be a "blip". This is one hell of a blip.

...When the unexpected and inconceivable intrudes on life, and it will, deal with life's actual events – don't obsess about perceived eventualities. Relax – enjoy the ride.
Michael J. Fox – Oprah Magazine

Thanks Taxotere (Chemo drug)

My nails hurt. Typing this hurts. Please God don't let my nails come off.

I hope I don't get cancer again.

Obsessing Over Not Obsessing

I tend to obsess and I'm trying to stop. I came across the Michael J. Fox quote and it really spoke to me. Funny how sometimes life presents the things you need to know. I'm trying to be in the moment. I guess I have an issue with control. Raised by a single mother with emotional highs and lows, I held so much in and needed to feel I had command of my emotions. Some of the survival skills I learned no longer serve me well. They inhibit me from being present in my life with confidence and joy. I learned how to hold on real tight.

Today

I've become even more jealous of pretty girls than ever. I am totally unattractive now and I look at beautiful women out there and want to cry. I feel a yearning in my soul to feel pretty, carefree, happy, excited and not weighted down by cancer.

What I Know

The Ride

You will find new friends in unexpected places
You will forgive friends for not calling
You will forgive yourself for being unlike the You that you know
You will sleep
You will be angry
You will wish for the days before cancer
You will count your blessings
You will be scared
You will be uncomfortable
You will be brave
You will learn about your body
You will complain
You will feel like pitying yourself
You will find strength you didn't know you had
You will feel ugly
You will feel lucky
You will want to feel normal and you will find the new normal
You will learn to trust the medical team
You will be amazed at how well you do
You will zone out and watch hours of television
You will feel awkward
You will have a love-hate relationship with your wig
The days will be long but the months will go by quickly
Your nails will hurt
Your muscles will ache
Your children will go about their business
Your husband or partner will be there for you
Your family will check on you constantly
You will find humor
You will enjoy your favorite foods

You will be glad to have your taste buds back
You will discover a new you, mixed in with the old you
You will rediscover your hobbies
You will reveal your issues with your work associates
You will have long conversations with people and learn how
    much compassion there is
You will push yourself to get up in the morning
You will stay up late thinking a million thoughts
You will journal
You will still be scared of needles
You will learn to take comfort medicine
You will receive insurance bills in the mail
You will go to a support group
You will go to an event even though you feel conspicuous in your
    wig
You will use lots of moisturizer
You will cry a lot
You will learn to look at yourself in the mirror
You will accept the unknown
You will slow down
You will pat yourself on the back for getting through the simplest
    things
You will go shopping
You will do the dishes
You will procrastinate, like you did before
You will consider the "before" you, versus the "after" you
You will make a list of the many things you'd like to do
You will eliminate many unnecessary actions from your life
You will think about your childhood
You will be bloated
You will cry in the shower when your hair falls out
You will celebrate every single new hair that comes in
You will search the internet late into the night
You will feel incredibly lazy

You will watch happy people and take note of their light step

You will remember when you were one of those people

You will have flashbacks of the utter shock the moment you were
    told

You will decide who to tell and who not to tell

You will have new admiration for everyone who experienced this
    before you

You will cry when anything bad happens to anybody

You will want to feel strong

You will mourn the loss of your eyelashes

You will love yourself in new ways

You will forgive others for not knowing what to say

You will enjoy not having to spend time on your hair

You will spend more time putting on make-up

You will hug strangers who tell you their story

You will be told that you are doing so well

You will want to smile

You will look at "before" pictures of yourself and miss that person

You will always remember the date you started treatment

You will, surprisingly, not notice when you start to feel better but
    then be glad that you do

You will eat a lot of protein

You will think that every single person knows

You will find reasons to be happy

You will forgive people for their mistakes

You will look at people differently

You will be strong for your children

You will need quality sleep

You will eat chocolate

You will get hot flashes and finally understand what the fuss is
    about

Your head will get cold

You will walk the dog

You will continue to say please and thank you like you always have

You will be a little obsessed with your heart rate, blood pressure, blood work, weight

You will receive *a lot* of advice

You will try to take better care of yourself; there is always room for improvement

You will always wonder why this happened

You will push forward each day knowing how precious time is

You will feel small, like one tiny creature in a very large unpredictable universe

You will consider all of the things that have been meaningful to you

You will observe how other people's actions do matter

You will receive many wonderful greeting cards

You will have lots of Tylenol on hand

You will see the inside scoop in many medical settings; some of it will be fascinating, some of it will be terrifying, some of it will be frustrating

You will want to write a book

You will watch the holidays come and go and they will all be a mark in time during this phase of your life

You will envision your future

You will smile

You will wear your chemo hat and not give a damn

You will learn to wear a scarf on your head

You will want to be babied

You will go see a movie

You will seek humor

You will not sweat the small stuff

You will do your best to trust your instincts

You will wish you never had to go through any of this but you will be wiser for it

You will be jealous of healthy people

You will be jealous of beautiful flowing hair

You will look at people's eyelashes

You will become more aware of societal expectations in how we look and act

You will be wary of germs

You will question anything remotely toxic

You will read labels more

You will realize you cannot control everything

You will examine how you've conducted yourself throughout your life

You will wonder what you'd be remembered for

You will be glad to not have to shave

You will wash your hands frequently

You will plan your future

You will still get pissed off at stupid drivers

You will notice how many people around you are providing services that you need

You will admire the strength and achievements of others

You will learn to have patience with your body and the time it takes to heal

You will quit drinking coffee because it makes you jittery but then you will drink it again and enjoy it

You will feel emotional and overwhelmed

You will put certain things on hold

You will accomplish many things

You will see your children finish a year of school

You will celebrate other people's birthdays

You will discuss many ailments with your doctors

You will want to escape to a beautiful island

You will find the resolve to keep going

You will indulge

You will treat yourself with kindness

You will have enormous compassion for others

You will think back to all of the people you've known who went through this

You will be incredibly grateful for medical advances

You will feel incredibly sad for those who are gone because
   medicine couldn't help them

You will learn how different each person is and why we make the
   choices we do

You will be grateful for your arms, legs, eyes, nose, mouth, ears,
   muscles, brain, fingers, toes

You will take your wig off on a hot summer night

You will dream about having hair

You will dream about having eyelashes

You will learn about the wig industry

You will feel guilty for the high cost of having a disease

You will feel somewhat tarnished by this intruder in your life

You will realize you are human

You will wish you could stop thinking about it

You will be tired of talking about it but you will feel compelled
   if anyone asks the simplest question

You will be so, so happy on your last day of chemo then you will
   be so, so sad when you have to recover from that last one and
   it takes longer than you thought it would and you will wish
   your hair could magically reappear

You will wonder if you should have done the Penguin Cold Cap
   to preserve your hair

You will be shocked at the cost of wigs, supplements, skin care

You will learn to accept your situation

You will be more and more grateful for all of the good things
   you've ever experienced

You will enjoy the sunshine

You will still enjoy the rain

You will allow others to take care of you

You will be shocked by how many people have or are going
   through this

You will make lists so you don't forget stuff

You will still forget stuff

You will rest

You will play music in your car really loud

You will feel like a science experiment

You will turn the air conditioner on and off in your car constantly

You will actually watch daytime television and enjoy it

You will give yourself permission to feel like total crap

You will garden

You will remember all of the good times

You will discover the many uses for wig tape

You will read

You will remember to back up your computer files

You will get to know many of the nurses at the oncology office

You will meet a surgeon

You will ask questions

You will follow doctors' orders and not eat food from a salad bar, or eat sushi, just to be safe

You will gain water weight

You will at first be annoyed at the time it takes to go to so many doctor appointments and treatments but you will come to appreciate that it is to make you well

You will meet other bald people

You will see how brave people are

You will cry thinking that other people might see you that way even though you don't feel brave at all

You will feel vulnerable

You will have many prescriptions

You will make sure to sleep with your favorite pillow

You will have a temporary handicap placard which makes you feel awful until you start using it at metered parking, and then appreciate it

You will see sick people

You will see young sick people

You will see old sick people

You will remember all of your favorite songs

You will argue with your daughter

You will laugh with your kids

You will go out to dinner

You will get rashes, possibly a sty, constipation, diarrhea, fatigue, muscle aches; it will all go away

You will want to run in the next cancer marathon

You can't help but stare at women's breasts

You will buy too many hats

You will lose your body hair even in your nose

You will receive many texts from people wishing you well

People will send food

You will walk on the beach

You will receive phone calls from doctors and your heart will skip a beat every time the phone numbers show up on the caller ID

You will eat soup

Your mouth will be sensitive

You will actually laugh

You will have normal days

You will run errands

You will exercise

You will plan celebrations for getting through each thing

You will get extremely emotional seeing anything on the internet about survival

You will like to hear the good stories of people who survived this

You will have a deep sadness, even for those you have never met, if they did not make it

You will learn how to deal with fear

You will learn that you can function despite it all

You will recover from surgery

You will have intense anxiety before surgery

You will be thankful for all of the nurses who are so amazing and treat you with such kindness

You will be scared to look at the incision site

You will read the post-op instructions

You will enjoy a good meal the day after surgery

You will sleep in as late as you please

You will be glad to see the sunshine

You will put water in the dog's bowl

You will pee blue from the pre-surgery dye injected into the incision sites

You might be told that you need more surgery

You might lose one or both of your breasts

But you will realize that you are not your breasts. You are you.

You are still the same person with the same hopes and dreams

You still love animals and chocolate and hearing the birds chirp in the morning

You will want to celebrate the milestone of having gotten through so much

You will wake up one morning and realize how strong you feel, and how great that is, and you will want to tell the world to not sweat the small stuff and don't be cranky. Just jump for joy!

You will receive get well flowers and enjoy them immensely

You will love yourself more than ever before.

We'll Now Be Inserting Two Wires into Your Breast
Or
Are You F***ing Kidding Me?

I am not brave. When fear creeps in I think about my children, or smelling a flower, or looking at a beautiful blue sky, or walking my dog or watching a great movie. I think about the life I wish to have, the trips I want to take with my husband.

I have lost my innocence. I've been forced to contort my body in ways during various procedures. Wire localization comes to mind.

Let's talk about Wire Localization for a moment shall we?

This is a procedure done immediately before the lumpectomy.

The mammogram locates the small titanium clips that were placed in the breast during the biopsy. Once the clips are seen, a thin wire is placed in the breast and sticks out about two or three inches. I presumed procedures like this were a thing of the past. I was wrong. Some women apparently faint from this one. The wire marks the spot where the surgeon will remove the tissue (and some surrounding healthy tissue) that might not be palpable after treatment, as in my case.

I had two lumps. One very, very small – slightly smaller than a pea – under the nipple. The other lump was larger, more like a grape. As we know the smaller of the two caused me quite a bit of pain during the biopsy because there are so many nerve endings there. I gave the doctors a heads up as we began the wire procedure. I had to brace myself yet again. The numbing shot is actually what hurts. The doctor cleverly dealt with the less painful lower area first so the work could be done as efficiently as possible. The mammogram procedure itself is awkward but this is the world we live in.

It was time to numb the smaller area. I sat in a chair (because standing could result in fainting) and faced the mammogram monster. The injection went in. I had hoped I'd get away with it that time. But no. The piercing pain radiated throughout my breast and crawled all over my body. I trembled from head to toe. Ah, but I had to hold still for the mammogram. I cried without breathing like a baby that wails silently and turns purple. The doctor and nurses in the room (there were three people total) took a step back and reminded me to breathe. I finally did. The second wire was placed. There were two wires sticking out of my breast covered in gauze. Then I had to wait for a wheelchair to arrive to roll me over to surgery. The wait was longer than anticipated. I was put in a little room. I was shaking. The numbing was wearing off and I felt the wires. Once again Chuck was waiting for me. His first question to the nurse was if I was in pain. All I could do was nod my head. Yes, there had been pain. But it passed. All of the discomforts were temporary.

The attendant wheeled me over to surgery while Chuck walked alongside. I had wondered why I needed to be awake for this charming wire procedure. Someone explained to me that it is typically a quick process (even though it feels like an eternity) and because I was about to be given general anesthesia during the lumpectomy this is how it's done. I wish they could have knocked me out for this one.

This procedure was one of the highlights of my entire breast cancer experience. There has got to be a better way. The only thing I can say is that my case had the bad luck of a tumor located in an extremely sensitive spot. That's the way it goes sometimes.

Although I cannot possibly imagine what women went through many years ago when technology was less advanced, I think there is much work to be done. Someone must come up with a better machine than the current mammogram equipment. We need a Dyson mammogram machine. (I wonder if he'd consider it. Take a look at my letter at the beginning of this book and let me know what you think.)

I'm glad that chemotherapy has dramatically improved. My oncologist had even said "We don't let you puke." It is still a tough experience but tolerable most of the time. Even if I had some queasiness I was armed with medicine just in case. The trick is to get ahead of it and stop nausea in its tracks. As the oncology team said, "It's like getting the flu every three weeks for a few months". Great.

But this wire localization ordeal should win an award for one of the most emotionally derailing experiences ever. Not every breast cancer patient goes through this, so that's a plus. It felt pretty undignified to me even post chemo which is maddening to begin with. Not to mention feeling anxious as I was about to go into a procedure to remove breast tissue.

Staying Strong

Five Days

I have gotten used to the waiting game. Or so I thought. Woke up this morning and felt weak in the pit of my stomach anticipating news from the surgeon. I am hopeful that she got clear margins and the lumpectomy was successful but there is no way to be sure until the pathology report comes back.

I have gotten used to bracing myself for news. Each time is hard. Waiting for the first biopsy result was hard. The second biopsy report on the right breast was nerve wracking. Waiting for the MRI result was less worrisome because we knew the tumors had shrunk. That was a definite highlight as it had turned out so well.

And now this. The surgery report. The sentinel node. The breast tissue. It all needs to come back with no evidence of cancer. What if there is one bad cell in there? How do they know? I guess that is why I have to go through radiation, Herceptin and Tamoxifen. That is why. Today is Wednesday. I should hear no later than this Friday. These next few days are harder than I thought.

Nothing Is What It Seems

Sentinal node okay. No cancerous lymph nodes. But surgical margins too close. Now what? Another surgery, but what? Don't know. Very disappointing. Very difficult emotionally. Thank God for support group. Seeing plastic surgeon on Monday. Have to remember my life has been saved. Have to be grateful for the doctors. I have been through chemo. I have done it. I hate the word "mastectomy". Didn't think I'd have to go down that road. Re-excision (more tissue removal) would be preferred. Don't know what is next.

Celebrating my daughter's 14th birthday this weekend. I should enjoy being a mom for a few days.

I'm Still Alive

But I must now go through surgery to remove my breast because going back in to remove more tissue from my "A" cup would leave me with a de-constructed breast. So the solution is a mastectomy to be sure they get it all. What an awful thing. It is so very sad but my life is more important than one small breast. I will most likely have reconstruction using my abdominal tissue. It is hard to realize this new truth as I sit here calmly typing this while the television is on, the breeze is blowing, the dog is resting. Hard to believe that I will be put through a ten-hour surgery. Yes it is my choice to do this rather than an implant or no reconstruction at all. This is what I want. I learned that an implant has to be replaced in ten or fifteen years and I'd rather not deal with that.

This is not easy and I must be kind to myself. I must try not to hold on too tight. I should do things that make me happy. What else can I do?

Had Herceptin infusion today. One more thing to be grateful for. It is hard these days to hold on to hope. I had hoped the lumpectomy would save my breast. But it could not.

I am sad and will miss my breast. I will miss having sensation on that breast. I will miss seeing my natural body and am filled with dread anticipating all of the scars.

I must slow down and get myself through each day. Just each day. That is all I have to do. I don't have to be anxious about tomorrow. I don't have to worry if I'm doing something wrong or if I don't get everything done in one day. I must love myself. It is hard to push away the feelings of extraordinary guilt for what I am putting Chuck through.

How Many Breasts Will You Be Ordering Today?

Tissue from my abdomen will create a new breast. The compromise is a scar from hip to hip on my lower abdomen. Surgeon says it is a good decision, that the result will be excellent. The what-if-I-get-cancer-again question is a tough one. I don't know if I can ever get a perfect answer. The surgeon's office will call with suggested dates for after Chuck's birthday.

I am trying not to over think and trust my gut instinct based on the information I have been given by my doctors. Facing each day, each challenge, each thought, each movement with some amount of love for myself. Trying not to guilt myself for whatever it is I don't get right these days. Forgiving myself.

A Precious New Life

My sister is five days away from giving birth to her first child. We are both in an anticipatory state of mind. How incredible that she and I are both going through life-changing events days apart.

My mastectomy is scheduled for September twenty. I am doing my best to be at peace with it. Preparing myself emotionally as best I can. Will go to support group tomorrow. Wish I didn't have to feel pain and be unable to tend to the kids, the house, the dog, my usual life. Instead I will be drugged and physically manipulated.

I must presume I will live. That I am on the upswing now. That the very worst is behind me. That I can continue on, pursue the things I wish. See my children grow. Go places with Chuck. Eat good food. Enjoy ice cream and happiness.

I hope the birth of my niece is a good sign. A sign that everything will be alright. I must trust. I must be positive. I must forge ahead. I must keep on.

New Fear

Ten Days Before My Mastectomy

Time

My watch stopped working about a month ago, maybe longer. Has time stood still? Is it some strange sign that the watch I have worn for well over a decade has stopped working right at the same time my life has been at risk? Does it mean that somehow my watch has slowed to a stop to allow me to heal? Or does it mean that time has stopped because I am sick and can no longer move forward? I don't believe that second one. I am not sick, not really. We all have cells with potential for illness. The cells that created those two lumps have been removed.

Perhaps time has stopped so that I can learn to slow down. I can let myself heal without worry of time. Yes that is it. My universe is not concerned with exacting deadlines. Not so much. Not now. My body, my living, breathing body, with all of its intricate detail, needs every minute of every day to heal. In ten days my body will be assaulted by brilliant surgeons who will take me apart and put me back together, reconstructing what nature made. And then I will heal again. I will not need a watch.

The minutes will turn into hours, the hours into days, the days into weeks, until finally, I will have this last excruciating step behind me. Unless I need radiation. Then I'll need more minutes, more hours, more days. Perhaps time has stopped because my watch is not capable of handling this one. It is bigger than one calendar day. It is bigger than one appointment to the next.

My watch on my wrist was overpowered by the forces of the universe that brought me to these days. No need to keep track of time. Useless. Like when I would go on trips with my dad and we would take off our watches. Vacation wasn't about keeping track of time the way we normally would. But I feel naked without the watch on my wrist. Even though I keep track of time on my phone or computer or microwave at home, my watch has been my definitive guide. When I leave the house I feel the empty space where my watch should be. I feel as though I am dangling over some unknown space. And that is exactly what I am doing. This unknown space ten days before a major surgery unlike anything I have ever experienced before. This space between cancer and hopeful cure. This space between hair loss and hair re-growth. This space between devastation of the awful news and the journey back to the joy of being alive. My watch knows. It quit on me to tell me to never mind the minutes, the hours, the days. To look beyond those measures. To value the bigger picture; the magnitude of saving my life. The enormity of so many minutes, hours and days that will be added to my life, thanks to my doctors, and my husband who has so much patience no time keeper could possible measure. It is so big, my watch could not handle it.

The truth is the battery had repeatedly failed the last couple of years. But isn't that interesting. The oncologist said the tumors were brewing the last two to three years leading to the point of detection. My watch knew. My watch had reliably told me where I was in my day for so many years until recently when the battery kept failing, trying to tell me to stop, to listen, to watch, to feel. But I didn't know.

I looked at watches at a store the other day. The emptiness of no watch on my wrist has felt almost like an unfinished story, opportunity missed, a void. So I gave into the feeling and enjoyed looking at sparkling new watches. Like new hope. Like a new beginning. So many styles. I saw some I liked. I was going to ask to see some but the one sales person around got busy with another customer and I realized it wasn't time yet. It wasn't time to pay attention to time. The customer was taking quite a while and I did hang around hoping he'd finish up. But time told me to wait. To let it go. To not concern myself with the minutes, the hours, the days. That my life now, this journey I have been on, this experience, is bigger than time. Bigger than a day. That I must learn to measure by faith, by feeling, by gratitude. By the waves inside of me that flow until the tears come out.

When I have healed from this place I will buy a new watch. A new device to keep track of my new time. My second chance. My new measure of my life. I had the same watch for over a decade. A lovely Bulova that went with everything. It sits now, on my desk, motionless. Still. Waiting. Waiting for me to say goodbye to the old time. I re-set the time the other day to see how long it would run. It ticked for about half an hour and stopped again. When I inquired at the watch store when it had first failed they said it would cost $95 to repair. So it wasn't worth fixing. But I am. I am worth fixing. My watch served me well for many years. The truth is, in the last five years I haven't been able to see the tiny calendar date number. I can explore a new style, a new measure of time. My new watch and I will hopefully be together for a very long time. That is my goal. For now time doesn't own me and I am free to ride the wave. To let go of conventional time and find direction from within. The sun guides me every day. I don't need a watch to tell me that I am alive.

Night-time is the hardest. I am afraid of letting go as the sky darkens. I am afraid of going to sleep, of letting time slip away. My eyes get weary though and with the help of homeopathic sleep aids, I get rest. Sure enough the sun rises again. And here I am. Without my watch. Without the ticking. Without the mark on my wrist that has propelled me forward for so many years.

My new watch will be a new mark in time. The next chapter. The minutes, the hours, the days, of the next parts of my story.

Goodbye Left Breast

It must be true that one's state of mind has something to do with the outcome and even the reactions to drugs. You do have to disconnect from your own body a little bit to tolerate the medical manipulation that surrounds you. You have to give your body over to the people who have been trained to take care of it. I am in awe of those people. The body is after all, just a living organism. If you remove the thoughts and emotions from the body itself it is easy to see how doctors approach it. Then there is pain of course. Pain changes a person. But it is momentary. It is temporary. There are drugs for pain.

Tomorrow I will have the mastectomy. I know I will be well taken care of. I have such respect for all of the doctors and staff.

I am not brave. I am not remarkable. I simply wish to live.

Recovery and Love

Coming Home

"Toooo hottt, howww lonnngg" were my first words out of the twelve hour surgery. It took that long because first the breast surgeon performed the mastectomy and then the plastic surgeon removed abdominal tissue and arteries, and then painstakingly re-attached it to form a new breast. And that's for one breast. The first forty-eight hours after surgery were crucial to be sure the re-attached blood vessels were functioning. Nurses came in and checked on me every two hours those first couple of days. There is no rest in hospitals!

Apparently I repeated my "how long" question three or four times and the nurse explained that I had a warming blanket over me. Well that blanket was very hot.

On day three I awoke to the sound of my own heavy breathing and my heart beating hard and fast in my chest. I was coming out of a dream that felt more like a nightmare. I had been searching for my daughter but instead found a small dog that had a human facial expression, staring up at me from the ground. My Rabbi appeared and I asked him to help me find my daughter. He said he knew where she was and that I should follow him. We walked along a dirt path that looked like a foreign country. It all seemed terrifying for some reason and I awoke with a feeling of desperation.

Exactly at the moment my eyes opened, my mother was entering my hospital room and she saw me crying, all alone in my bed with no one around. I cried out and told her to please get a nurse because I felt that something was terribly wrong. She came to the side of the bed, her face almost touching mine, stroked my fuzzy head and said "It's alright sweetheart. Everything is alright". I could see there were tears in her eyes but I could also feel her sense of purpose in helping me get a grip on the moment. I wanted my blood pressure checked because I felt like my chest was going to burst. A nurse came in and assured me that I was okay. I calmed down and understood that I was recovering from twelve hours on anesthesia and pain meds pumping through me.

On the morning of day four I was told it was time to go home. I looked at the doctor as though he was totally insane. Sure enough later that day I was ready. There was a strange quiet after my family had all gone and my husband and I waited for the wheelchair. We surveyed the room one last time like we do at a hotel to be sure nothing was left behind. I was finally going home.

Those four days I knew nothing of the outside world. We arrived at the garage level and there were people; people living their lives as I was wheeled back into my former life. The vantage point from the wheelchair was low and I watched the cars come and go. Finally our black Prius arrived. I was finally going home.

Someone opened the door for me and I carefully made my way into our car. The world was out there waiting. We left the garage and I saw the glow of the afternoon sun. I was still woozy from days on drugs. The little ride from Westwood to Santa Monica felt precarious.

We arrived at our front door. I was home. Everything was the same. I had wondered if I'd have the strength to walk by myself to the bedroom. I looked down the hall and realized it was easy. I said a brief hello to the kids and I went to go lay down for what turned out to be a three-hour nap.

Today is the first day I am alone for a little while. I am home with myself and my thoughts. All is quiet like any other day. A friend will be here soon. I still have one drain in place on the right side of the abdominal incision, which looks like I have a tennis ball in my pocket. And I can't stand up straight. I walk leaning forward like a little old lady. I don't want to look sick. I want to look and be well. I'm working on eating well.

I am home, each day looking brighter.

The Show Must Go On

I had thought long and hard about when to tell my client about my situation. It was a large project for a law firm and once I was diagnosed I did not pursue additional work. My oncologist had told me that most people work through all or most of chemotherapy and I felt confident I could do it. I proceeded with caution knowing that if I had to tell the client, I would.

As the weeks went on I saw that I was perfectly capable of emailing back and forth with my client and visiting showrooms to source furniture selections. I had energy and was thinking clearly. I was completely up to the task and I was thrilled to have the work. What made life a little easier was that this particular client was not in a rush. In fact, they had some delays in decision making which would have normally caused me some frustration, but turned out to be a blessing. The delays allowed extra time for rest and did not compromise my responsibilities.

I continued to source carpet, furniture and fabric options, specify paint colors, and met with my client only a few times during the months of chemotherapy.

Once the three and a half months of chemo were done and I was headed toward my first surgery, I decided it was time to tell. I had tremendous anxiety anticipating the conversation and had drafted a few emails that I wound up not sending. I was in a meeting reviewing the project timeline and finalizing fabric samples when I decided I couldn't hide it any longer. I had been wearing my wig for some time of course, and unless my client was being polite, she seemed genuinely shocked when I told her the news. And a little bit impressed. I had gotten through so much and there I was, fully functional. Even with an excellent prognosis it was difficult to share my news. Although I felt constantly on the verge of tears, I didn't cry. I said "I need to let you know that I've been treated for cancer and have recently finished chemo. And this is a wig". My client looked at me and said "Wow". Of course she offered her sincerest wishes for my recovery. The ripple effect of my illness had reached every corner of my life. There I was, telling this person I hardly knew that I was going through breast cancer. I was relieved I had let the cat out of the bag. Rather than feeling undermined by my vulnerability, I felt I could move forward honestly and handle whatever came next. After my lumpectomy I received the most beautiful flowers from the firm.

The amazing thing is, this law firm represents clients who have contracted diseases such as cancer, lung disease and other serious ailments associated with toxicity in their environments. Of all clients in the whole wide world, I was providing design services for a law office that fought for those affected by life-threatening illness. It was ironic and a blessing that I had that job at that time. And I was grateful for their understanding and compassion. I continued working on the project until my reconstruction surgery, at which point I notified them that I would be recovering for a few weeks. Their assistant coordinated with me on the remaining tasks.

The 10,000 square foot office space was painted in warm neutrals. Old teal colored carpet was removed and new carpeting in a contemporary pattern was installed, energy efficient solar blinds were hung in every window, and new ergonomic chairs and media consoles in a stunning walnut finish updated the conference rooms.

Any project I have ever worked on, and especially one which requires coordination of many trades such as flooring installers, custom furniture orders, and painters, requires deft communication. I was grateful support was in place to complete the project.

I hadn't wanted stupid cancer to get in the way. But as the days unfolded during those months, it was ultimately out of my control and required new (scary) conversations, and new ways of thinking.

Music

I decided to play some music this morning. It was time to play Beethoven. But it wasn't with my other CDs. Then I remembered I had put it in my nutrition folder prior to surgery as I've been keeping track of how to best fortify my body during chemo and healing.

I had left a note on the CD cover that says *"If I don't make it, play this entire album at my funeral"*.

The music is something I discovered long ago in the records my mom had after she and my father divorced when I was a little girl. The album, Moonlight Pathetique & Appassionata Sontas, has been my all time favorite classical music my entire life. I have played it over and over again. It has brought me to tears every time. If I were blind this music would help me see. This music encompasses every human emotion. I felt that if I had died in the operating room this music would express everything I could hope to express; the range of emotions as a young child, young adult, young mother, and beyond into my more mature years. This music has been there for me. I was scared of dying during surgery. I didn't think I would but fear crept in at night leading up to the big day.

I was delighted that I remembered where I had put the CD and saw my note. Even though I did in fact survive the surgery, I think I will leave the note on the plastic case.

The physical and emotional challenges of the last nine months were impossible to imagine. But I am here. Now my body is healing from the ordeal of a twelve-hour surgery. It is giving me a chance to pause and listen to what I feel. I had forgotten about music. Finally I was ready to listen again.

It also takes me away from dwelling on the slow process of getting better. It takes me out of my head and into a different place. I blasted it loud and forgot about things for a while.

The next time I play it I'll be different than I am now. I'll have gotten through one more hurdle. I'll listen again with an open heart. Like hearing a bird on a spring day.

Home after Surgery

People think I bounce back well. But I have been brutalized. I have been through a cycle of healing for nine months. I know I'm not dying. I'm living. So much attention has been lavished upon me in the past two weeks. And now I am alone on this Saturday morning. It is good to be alive. How could anyone possibly consider this a blip?

I have one more drain to be removed from the right side on my abdomen.

I received the wonderful news that it is highly *unlikely* I'll need radiation. I would do it if my wonderful team of doctors said I should. But apparently I would not receive any additional benefit from it since cancer had not spread to my lymph nodes. So the mastectomy did what it should do.

Now I have a new breast in place of my original one. It is swollen and the entire area is bruised, deep purple, yellow and blue, so it is hard to know how it will look. Pressing on it, it feels soft and natural. I know I made the right choice to reconstruct. I've had so many drugs pumped into me I know my body and brain are going through a transition now. I know this intellectually. But the waves of emotion and exhaustion come over me without warning.

The abdominal incision is tight and I cannot stand up fully

straight yet. Soon I'll be all better. Not that long from now. I'm told it takes four weeks to heal. I must persist. I must be kind to myself. I must sleep when I need. In the not too distant future I'll be done with Herceptin and then have the port removed. Then I'll heal from that. Then I'll always have that scar. So many scars. Hopefully my husband will accept this new me.

You Cannot Do it Alone

It seems as though the strength of a thousand people cannot lift you from the despair. And yet when your family rallies around you, you do find the resources within. On the one hand you face it all with gusto. You immediately realize what your life means and you want to fight. I've always hated that word. But I understand it now. You want to fight and you do. It takes all of your strength. And when you have conquered each hurdle you feel stronger. But no, you cannot do it alone. Whoever those family members are, they are precious. They are there for you. They tell you that you can do it. They pray for you. Your friends want so much to make it go away. They send food. And they pray. All of the prayers add up. You need every one. I've never liked the word "fight" because it sounds so mean. But this cancer thing is not to be fooled with. And fight you will. It is a test of endurance over a long period of time. You find a place in your soul you never knew was there. You face your darkest thoughts. You consider your most precious moments. Sometimes it is hard to have the strength to even think at all. You cannot believe this is you, the person who is so self-sufficient. So able to do whatever needs doing. Now you need people. You need enormous amounts of comfort. Not pity. No. Just the comfort of knowing that positive energy surrounds you. Nothing else matters.

The battle never ends. You learn that you will always look over your shoulder. But you also decide what each day can be for you. As your hair returns and the color in your cheeks improves, you live again.

For now, caring people in my life hold me up. They have created a circle of love around me. The amount of courage I have had to summon is only equal to the amount of love and support I have received. The two are intertwined. You cannot do it alone. You cannot and should not hide. You must reach out and receive those prayers.

Thanks Mom

So many thoughts are running through my head. But at this moment I want to remember to thank my mom. After the big surgery, she was there for me. She was strong for me. I can't imagine how difficult it has been for her coming to follow-up appointments, watching me have drains removed, wincing in pain; to see my days unfold, witnessing the emotional roller-coaster that is this cancer thing.

We've had rough times but I was lucky she could be there for me. There is healing there for both of us. She really came through. Good things do happen.

Now What

The big fuss is over. Suddenly doctors don't need to see me as much. There is a strange quiet. The emergency is behind me.

Hair growing. No more chemo. No surgery for at least three months (to remove the port and add a nipple). All I need to deal with is Herceptin and Tamoxifen, which is no small beans, but still.

What I have achieved is a miracle. This wasn't in my plans. But it happened. The panic is less now. I am on a maintenance schedule. Waves of memories come to me every so often. But looking back is easier. The fear of chemo long gone. The aches and pains of the Neulasta shot, gone. No more rashes, fluid retention, hair loss. Waking up in the middle of the night contemplating if I can get through it all, subsiding fast.

Thoughts of the future are allowed to come in to focus. Now I must begin to muster the strength to live happily again. To assume the worst is behind me and to focus on what my life is about.

And I have eyelashes again. It's wonderful.

The Work of Getting Back to Work

My hair is a little longer than a boy's crew cut now. It lays flat and looks rather chic. I don't recognize the person I see in the mirror but I'm working on it.

As part of my membership in the American Society of Interior Designers I attend lectures for learning credits, usually held in showrooms, and I also go to events for fun. I receive invites regularly and have missed many this past year.

Yesterday one of my favorite interior designers, Barbara Barry, was having a book signing at Baker Furniture in West Hollywood for her new book *Around Beauty*. I decided that I needed to get my ass over there to kick start my inspiration going forward. I have always been a huge fan and this was my opportunity to meet her in person and get myself back into the real world of living.

I stood in line with her gorgeous new book in my hands and sat with her as she signed it *"To Alicia, a kindred spirit, Barbara, xo"*. I was thrilled to have met her.

As I sat with her for those few moments I told her I had always admired her work and that I had had a rough year pointing to my hair, and it meant so much for me to be there. She looked at me with surprise and tears welled up in her eyes. At first I wasn't going to say anything but I couldn't help it. I wanted her to know how much I valued meeting her at this particular time in my life. We took a picture together as she had done with admirers who stood in line before me.

I left the Baker showroom buzzing with happiness. In my "past life", I'm not sure I would have been so bold as to point directly to my vulnerability. But I know now more than ever that life is too precious to hold back. It's perfectly fine to be genuinely me.

Gratitude

My Dirty Birthday

Here we are, the beginning of November. My attention turns to the garden once again as the rain comes which helps new plants thrive here in California. Finally I bought new ground cover visualizing the work to be done; digging the holes and spaces necessary in between the pavers. I find the work tremendously satisfying but need to carve out the time knowing I'll be sweaty and exhausted afterward.

Today, my birthday, I planted again before my brunch celebration. It also happens to be the day we turned back the clocks so I had an extra hour. The work of gardening takes me out of my head. I have planted many types over the years and sometimes success comes with little effort. Other times, despite tender loving care, a plant fails. Conditions have to be right.

Little did I know, last November my plants would die and I would face my own mortality. In the quiet of those hard, cold months, I pressed on. I finally have the energy again to enjoy the work, finally ready to put my gardening gloves on and get out the digging tools. I'm ready to pay attention to watering new plants and let nature take over. With care I will water and prune as needed. I will live this season in a place of gratitude and growth.

The Beauty of a Bad Situation

I breast fed child number one for about eight months, child number two for about five months. I was glad to breast feed although it can be rather isolating. It can be an intense time for a mother but rewarding nonetheless. In between early motherhood I worked on and off. Mostly though, I was home with our kids during their early years. I loved being a mom (I say with nostalgia and convenient memory loss of all of those diapers and messes, thank you). My hair in a ponytail for years, we read stories together, painted in the kitchen and sometimes in the front yard, picked flowers, played with clay and danced to music. These are the wonderful memories I get to keep. The crying, whining, cleaning, chasing, and negotiating all take a back seat to the joy of watching these miracles grow into actual people.

Little did I know my breast would betray me all these years later. The same breast that sustained the life of both of my children would develop this horrible life-threatening disease. Still, I am blessed. My body served an incredible purpose. To carry life, and to sustain it.

The past year has been a test for our family on so many levels. My maternal instincts want to shield my children from the awful trauma of watching me go through this ordeal. Now in their teens they will remember these days. My cancer will be part of their story. It breaks my heart.

It is my hope and belief that the years I shared with them when they were silly, adorable little kids dancing in our living room have paid off and that they are secure enough in their hearts and minds to navigate the difficult times.

Someday we'll look back and express to each other what is, at this moment, too dark, too unimaginable to unravel. In emergency mode there is no time to think. In emergency mode all energy must be focused.

Sometimes I still get lost muddling my way through the aftermath of what it took to save my life. All I need is to picture those two teenagers I live with and I am back on my path. Thankfully there are other pieces of my life that are coming back together.

I wish I could forever shelter my kids from illness and tragedy. I know I cannot. Instead I can offer tools to help handle what life deals us. Perhaps it makes us closer. Perhaps they will later understand that even on the precipice of loss there is still hope, ability, beauty and vision. There are gifts even in bad situations.

Our kids have seen family and friends support us through this unbelievable time. I hope that these are some of the memories they will take with them as they grow and mature and remember what mom went through that one crazy year. The election year. The year my daughter started high school. The year my son went to Israel. The year my niece was born. The year we all had a chance to acknowledge how blessed we are despite the unknown, despite the fear, the hats and wigs and quiet days of pulling together all of the necessary strength.

Despite it all they have been loved. I guess I couldn't ask for anything more than for my beautiful teenagers to feel loved. One day without breaking down into a fit of tears I can explain to them how much they helped me and gave me strength just by being themselves. The sheer joy it gives on my worst of days, watching these two kids come home from school, who multitask, texting while doing their homework (with music on in the background and maybe even TV too, while eating cookies). These beautiful teenagers who I get to live with are the greatest gifts and have fueled my fight each and every day. This is what they can know. This is all they need to know.

Looking Back, Looking Forward

Conversation with people always turns to what I've been through this past year. Especially because of the short hair it comes up.

There is still so much work to be done. I will receive Herceptin intravenously until January. I must process what I've been through while being a mom, a wife, a friend, a sister, a daughter, a business owner. I just want to breathe.

Tamoxifen

Despite my terrible fear of this drug I took my first pill today. Today is the first day of my life for the next five years. I hate the hot flashes due to "chemopause" which will continue thanks to this synthetic estrogen inhibitor. I would also like to not get blood clots or uterine cancer which are the known (although rare) risks of Tamoxifen. I do not want to be huddled down in this cancer story. But here I am. My mind is in fact starting to absorb other non-cancer things. It takes effort. Ultimately I think this is a huge learning curve. What else can it be?

At Peace with Life as I Know it

I am beginning to accept the feeling of vulnerability that comes with a cancer diagnosis. I'll never be perfectly comfortable with it. But maybe I can work with it. Maybe I can incorporate it into my life in a non-threatening way. Maybe I can embrace change. It sounds so simplified. Rather, my life has been amplified. I continue to process the impact. I feel the push and pull of fear and exuberance.

The Most Touching Email I've Ever Received
(from a close family member)

Was writing about you the other day, and realized something strange but wonderful. When you got sick I was in the deep throes of depression. Somehow seeing you go through this, trying so hard to stand by your side while I was so far away, well it helped me want to live again, watching you fight so hard. It gave me back a sense of hopefulness, willing you to be better made me in a way better. Bizarre, right? Perhaps, because what I was feeling was so self-indulgent and what you were going through was so incredibly real and terrifying it was like a slap in the face that I needed. But how do you say to someone thank you for fighting so gallantly for your life and in so doing giving me back mine? I guess just like that. Thank you. I love you always.

My Sweater

It is feeling very much like winter. Thanksgiving is coming soon. There is a distinct chill in the air and last night it rained. The sun tried to peak out but mostly today and yesterday the air is brisk at night and warm during the day.

Now I'm back to winter clothes. I must also deal with hot flashes. Layering is key. I made some good purchases last year that are serving me well. I have seen this thing through from one season all the way around the world to the same season again. That is how long this has been. This thing. It doesn't start and stop. Each step is a process. The day of diagnosis doesn't even come first. First there is suspicion. Then a follow-up. Then another test. Then more follow-up. Then a procedure, a result, a decision, a plan. Somewhere in there is the day of diagnosis which sets off a series of actions that are each distinct and strange. It all adds up to a continuation of figuring out this new territory. It is a gradual process in and out of doctor appointments and family discussions. In and out of emotions that are all strange and new, and terrifying.

I shuffle my sweaters around a little bit after finding some I had forgotten. I pull one out that I had not liked much before and hardly wore. This time I think, hey, this could work. It's a simple winter white crew neck. I decide it will go very well with my new pants. I'm so pleased to pull this sweater off of the shelf, like finding a dollar in a pocket from who knows when.

I pull it out from the shelf and see one long, silky brown hair against the white fabric. It is my hair from last winter. A long, lonesome strand. I pick it up and see the bronze tone in the light. I haven't used a blow dryer in almost a year. So here I am with my new short hair, finally at peace with it, and I stumble upon this remnant of me; one thin sliver from the past. I picked it off of the sweater and let it float away.

We Can Rebuild Her

It's been two months since the reconstruction on the left trouble-maker. I'm glad I did the surgery. I knew it was the right choice for me. But boy was I terrified. It took twelve hours to perform the mastectomy and then reconstruct, re-attaching the blood vessels. It's pretty fascinating stuff. I'm still getting used to the results. The new one feels very natural. There was never much pain with the exception of removing the drains. The abdominal area is still sensitive but no big deal. I hardly think about any of this during the course of my day.

About one month after the surgery at my follow-up with my plastic surgeon, my doctor admired his work. I have healed well and he was quite pleased. He took some photos (neck down) and we chatted about the whole experience and how grateful I am to have gotten through so much and how it's all looking pretty good. At some point toward the end of our friendly get-together

I asked about our next steps. He said, "This is not about cancer anymore, it is all elective now". Oh, I thought, well, that's true. There were no balloons. There were no noisemakers. There were no "hip, hip, hoorays". I stood there in the bright lights of my doctor's office processing this lovely little moment. (Our next steps involve a tattoo to replicate the areola.)

I got dressed and scheduled my next follow-up for three months later. My new boob and I left the doctor's office that day free to move about the world. Free to go on living.

Although there have been extraordinarily difficult moments up to this point, I am grateful. Taking a shower is still an emotional process. It is in that quiet space that I face my reality. Each day I am farther away from where this all began and closer to a new and better place.

I'm Trying

I really want to find the funny. I read other cancer blogs and there is humor. I think, why can't I be funny? I'm not sad twenty-four hours a day. Of course I laugh. Of course I appreciate every day. But I don't feel the joy. I get sad. People keep saying, *it's great the worst is behind you*. It implies that I am back to normal now. Okay, cancer gone, get to work!

I have a mammogram scheduled for the "good girl" (my healthy breast) on Monday. Scared. Most likely everything will be fine. I hate to think of any other possibility. I mean it wasn't supposed to happen in the first place right? So anything is possible. I have to prepare myself for that. I get paralyzed with fear. And my brain gets all muddled. So I spend too much time working my way around how I feel because it's too scary. I'm sick of it.

Can I live like this the rest of my life?

I could always have the other breast removed. Then I'd have

to get an implant. I didn't want implants. That is why I did the abdominal surgery but there was only enough tissue for one small breast. Here I am already conjuring getting rid of the good one and living with two fake boobs, both different from each other. It's total insanity. I am a total experiment.

Getting all worked up about this could not possibly be productive. But I want to be prepared. I have to distract myself from thinking about this any further. But I'm getting angry. Maybe angry is good. It forces me to have the adrenalin I need to keep going.

Can I Exhale Now?

Mammogram done and all is well. Relief.

We are all on different pages of the same story. We are all women taking care of our bodies. Our breasts, which start off innocently enough, become part of our young lives, and whether we realize it or not, our self-image.

I thanked the doctor for taking the time to look at my exam and giving me the result right away and I shed one tear of happy. I left the appointment and the thought popped into my head that sometimes mammograms are wrong. I called Chuck who was eagerly awaiting the good news and he tells me I have to stop torturing myself. He is right. I need to celebrate. My right breast, at this moment is healthy, and my left substitute breast is fine. I'm allowed to be happy. I can enjoy the holidays now.

I'm going for at least forty more holiday seasons. At least.

My Dog

Now that my kids are teenagers it's nice to hold my little poodle in place of a cuddly baby. I admit it, it helps. Our little poodle is pretty cute. He loves to sleep on someone's lap as long as they will allow it. He stares me down when I leave the house like I'm turning my back on my best friend. And when I come home we start all over again. He's only six pounds. He's the first dog our family has ever had. The main reason he is in our lives is that my daughter pleaded her case for two years straight. She was all of eight or nine years old but she was persistent.

She says she favors the cat more now. Not sure why. He is far less predictable and much more likely to bite or scratch.

That poodle has been such comfort. No matter if I was exhausted from the ordeal of treatment or surgery, he was there by my side. He follows me around the house. I'm sure he has helped bring my heart rate down when I was in moments of panic. I am so grateful for this little guy. My daughter thinks I'm crazy because I talk to the dog like he's a little person. But I swear he understands. He gives me great comfort. Animals do that. I think anyone suffering from any issue should have a dog. A loving, sweet, dog. I owe him nothing more than a walk and a biscuit. We don't have to talk about how I feel. We can just be. Together.

To Pray

I believe that every human being has prayed at one time or another.

Prayer is intention.

Prayer is silence.

It is

Imagination

Courage

Humbling

Ephemeral

Musical

Clarifying

Strength

Fortitude

It is to want

To pray is to find the inner voice of truth. To have a specific goal and to bring it forward in the mind.

Wisdom

Don't Be So Negative and Other Interesting Advice

It is hard for the one diagnosed to have to deliver the news to others. I still dread telling people what I have been up to this past year if the subject should come up. I dread it mostly because it's a sad tale of woe, and it sucks. I didn't tell everyone (like the lady at the grocery store or neighbors I don't see very often) and some people think I had the nerve to get a cool, short hair cut.

No one deliberately says something hurtful to someone diagnosed with a disease. But sometimes it comes out and it's hard to stop. I could very well have said something stupid to a cancer patient. I have been the recipient of some strange remarks. Not all bad. Mostly powerful, encouraging comments of love and support. But it is amazing what a few shitty comments will do to the soul during such a fragile time. The amount of support needed cannot be underestimated. But how? In what ways? Words? Actions? Food? Gifts? A smile? Information? How do you support someone who is facing disease of their own body? What do you say? What do you not say?

In a world where quick tidbits of information are the norm, how do you behave when someone needs good, old-fashioned love? In a world of immediate gratification how do you express how much you care? And what if you are not even close to the person? What if it's just an acquaintance? When you learn someone you know is going through this perhaps it changes your own life. Perhaps dealing with the subject of illness and death becomes a lesson. It certainly is for the cancer patient. Each day can feel like an impossible mountain to climb.

Most people want to know what they can do. Accepting help is a lesson for Miss-I-Can-Do-It-All, and offering help (or a kind word) is always a good thing.

After surgery I was the recipient of some awesome help by

way of food delivery using the calendar on the Lotsa Helping Hands website. I didn't have to keep track of a thing. It was wonderful and I'm grateful. In the early days of shock and disbelief, each day is pretty fragile. It is so important to feed the soul. I made a conscious effort to watch funny movies, listen to my favorite music and during down time after surgery, I read books I had been meaning to get to. Keeping the mind active (and distracted) does wonders.

I was also the recipient of some interesting remarks (sometimes when I least expected it) and I've heard of some doozies by others.

Here, I offer my top 10 dos and don'ts.

Top 10 list of what not to say to your friend who has been diagnosed with cancer:

1. Don't be so negative. Maybe your hair won't fall out.
2. Do you really need to wear that "shmata" (wig) in the house? Isn't it hot?
3. I threw up after my mastectomy.
4. My peach fuzz hair fell out after my last chemo.
5. You know you shouldn't eat any sugar, right?
6. Don't use antiperspirant.
7. You must wake up every day and think you're in a terrible nightmare.
8. Do you feel awful?
9. I was shocked when I found out about you.
10. I'd go without a wig if it were me.

Top 10 list of things to say (or do):

1. Send a basket of food. No spices or grease. Healthy soup is a good one.
2. Send a thoughtful or humorous card. (I received many that I will always treasure.)

3. Talk about someone who is at least five years out and doing well.
4. Compliment on an article of clothing or piece of jewelry.
5. Tell the person you are thinking of them every day and sending positive thoughts in their direction.
6. Tell them you are visualizing their well-being and sending them love.
7. Give them a hug.
8. Put a date in your calendar to call them. And call them to say hi, or email them to say hi. (This sounds so simple but receiving a call or message is a wonderful connection during a time that feels so disconnected.)
9. Tell them something funny or recommend funny movies. (Cancer patients actually do laugh.)
10. Pray for them and tell them that you will.

Sometimes the patient doesn't even know what they need or want. And it is hard for family and friends to feel helpless. If you find you have said or done something unintentionally awkward (it's understandable), own it, and then do or say something better next time. There are many opportunities during the course of cancer treatment to create something positive. You can't talk away the actual disease but you can be loving. You can just listen. You can offer something (an invitation to a yoga class perhaps) and let that person decide if they wish to take you up on it. If they don't, do not despair. Whatever goodness you put out there is ultimately appreciated. You can add to that person's ability to get through each day. That is a gift worth giving.

(What is a shmata you ask? An old Yiddish word mainly used to describe a cheap, raggedy piece of clothing.)

When the Whole Thing Started

I researched wigs like it was a new career. I went to a number of places, asked lots of questions and tried on many styles. I created a hair folder on my computer. I proceeded in an organized fashion absorbing new information about an industry of which I knew nothing. It kept me distracted from the despair. I needed something productive to focus on. I went through some trial and error until I found the right one.

First I spent $100 at a local wig place right after I was diagnosed when I was feeling desperate. I imagined my hair was going to fall out overnight and I wanted to be prepared. But I realized it was too big on my head and I thought, who was I kidding? I bought another synthetic wig that wound up costing $600 and much to my chagrin I was never happy with it. The color was all wrong and it was also too big around my ears. I couldn't imagine going to a project meeting with either of these wigs, and that's when I knew I had to get something that fit my extra small head properly. I had tried many and thought they all looked ridiculous and was on the verge of a total breakdown over it.

Finally I met Amy Gibson, owner of Created Hair, who produced for me the most wonderful head of real hair in an extra small cap size, to fit my extra small head. I had agonized over the price tag which was going to be anywhere from $1,500-$2,500 and had waited a day or two before I told my husband about the new purchase because he thought I had worked all of this out already. I bought the wig and although insurance declined any reimbursement, I was delighted that I had finally found The One. Not only that, Amy was kind and compassionate and helped me every step of the way to get used to my new hair during such a strange time in my life. Her stylist adjusted the color and tailored the cut, and Amy took the time to show me how to wash and dry it so it would always look fantastic. Amy is a true leader in the world of wigs. Her own experience with alopecia taught me a new perspective. She happens to be gorgeous whether or not she's wearing a wig and frankly that was a revelation for me at the time. When I met her I knew I had discovered an amazing resource and a wonderful person! People wear wigs for many reasons. Although mine was temporary, our friendship continues.

By treatment number three, I was wearing new wig number three, over the little bit of hair I had left. I felt conspicuous at first. I felt everyone could tell. But eventually I began to love my little wig. It was my shelter. Thanks to that hair I could blend in at a movie theater. It was convenient I must say. Just plop on the hair and go. Fantastic.

I was aware of the Penguin Cold Cap which preserves the hair (on the head but not elsewhere), and had decided against it. One must sit with the cap during chemo and for an additional five hours afterward, for a total of eight hours! The cost is roughly $1,500 for a three-month chemotherapy treatment such as mine, which is pretty much what I wound up paying for my too-small-for-anyone-else wig. At the time of this writing the Penguin Cap is not covered by insurance. I didn't have it in me to go through a freezing cold cap on top of everything else. That said, I know a few women who used the Penguin Cap and although their hair thinned, it worked out well for them. Because it is still in trials in the United States, it is not widely used here. It is gaining traction though and perhaps with more studies it will be approved by insurance companies.

Once in a while I also wore "hat hair". This is an interesting invention. It is a band of hair but open on the top. It must be worn with a hat (unless you really do in fact want to look like a clown). The advantage to this thing is that it allows for some breathability on the top of the head, especially if worn with a lightweight hat. I actually went to a client meeting with that ridiculous hat hair and no one seemed to have a clue. I wore it while my nice wig was being colored, and it saved the day.

Final Herceptin

I realized a strange thing. I won't be taken care of by all of the wonderful nurses anymore. Ending Herceptin is great, don't get me wrong. But it is sort of a safety net, being checked every three weeks. Being cared for; blood drawn, temperature taken, weight checked, and discussion with nurses about my situation. It has been a safe place. A place I'd never want to be, but grateful to be there nonetheless. The nurses at UCLA oncology are incredible. They treat everyone so kindly. I have to say I guess I will miss them.

Next week is the final one. The last time I'll sit in one of those big chairs. The last time one of those bags of medicine will hang over me. I'm excited.

Merging Back in with the General Public

Any time I go somewhere I haven't been in a while I'm conscious that I look different. I feel different too. Some people don't recognize me. People look at me with slightly sad but hopeful eyes asking me how I'm doing, how I'm feeling. I give the generic answer "feeling good…" What should I say; that the hot flashes are miserable. That my brain is fuzzy sometimes. That I get sad when I least expect it. That I hate looking at my body. That I miss my previous eyelashes. That I have trouble falling asleep. That I get nauseous in the morning sometimes. That I feel like I've been through a personal war. That I fear the future. That I am tired of looking back and just want to take one small step at a time.

In casual conversation I don't say those things. But that's fine because it forces me to smile and just be grateful.

Don't Bother Me if You Stub Your Toe

This body of mine had to put up with quite a lot this past year. I thought having two c-sections was good enough. Thankfully I've never broken any bones. Had the flu maybe twice. But after chemotherapy, a lumpectomy, a mastectomy and reconstruction, I (like many other fighting sisters) have earned some bonus points in the "wait 'til you hear my story" department.

I would rather have gone to Italy.

As I went through the various steps, the obstacle course, the maze, the twists and turns, the complicated road that saved my life, I learned something new. I was in the cancer bubble; in a land of uncertainty and unknowns.

When the word "cancer" hovers over a conversation in the real world I believe it is out of kindness that most people tend to avoid talking about something difficult they might be going through. There is a natural reluctance to divulge any problem in their life thinking it may seem irrelevant.

But we all face varying degrees of tough times which help us learn to adapt to the next challenge. Little hardships and the lessons that follow or the big lessons (I'm actually human) all count toward our own personal learning curve (and the pain in the ass things that happen along the way). In conversation we can take turns. I'll tell you how I'm doing with this cancer situation and you can share with me that your washing machine is broken. It's okay (I'd be annoyed if my washing machine was broken too).

Just because I had to suffer a little more (okay, a lot more) than some people does not mean the stuff of life is diminished in importance. I guess I sweat the small stuff a little less after my recent adventure. But I would still have compassion for someone upset about something, or evaluating a career move, or concerned that their child has a cold, even while I was being treated for cancer. You know, the important stuff that life is about. The thoughts, decisions, and problem solving that make us who we are each day, who we become, and who we want to be.

I'm still absorbing the impact and distilling the multitude of details that became the focus of last year. I'm still growing my eyelashes back (nature is funny like that) and there are a couple of fun filled appointments with my plastic surgeon in the near future. It has been a great honor to receive care from the UCLA medical group. They are spectacular people.

Behind the curtain no one wants to see there are brilliant doctors, nurses and staff helping patients through the challenges. The conversations are guided with the utmost respect. If I was concerned about a side effect (which they had likely seen many times in other patients) like a funny rash, or constantly tearing eyes, I was treated as a real human being experiencing this weird thing for the first time.

Of course now a year later, it is easier to understand the learning curve back in the distance. I suppose I'm stronger (and wiser?) today. Most of all I'm so very grateful that the cancer bubble is beginning to lift far up enough into the atmosphere to not intrude on every waking moment.

Just don't come complaining to me if you should happen to stub your toe. You'll be A-OK. I promise.

Truth

Pot, Marijuana, Cannabis, Weed

It is important to talk about this. Last time I had done it, it had been decades earlier. Then this cancer thing happened. At first I ruled it out. I don't like smoking. Xanax has been helpful but it has a downside. When I stop taking it I get jittery and moody (and get a throbbing headache) thus feel I should keep taking it but I don't want to continue with a synthetic drug indefinitely.

Back to pot. I thought, well, it couldn't hurt. The anxiety alone even before treatment began was sickening and paralyzing.

I did consider acupuncture for about two seconds. I had tried it a couple of times many years ago for muscle pain but the thought of lying down on a table being stuck all over the place didn't sound appealing. It's not my thing although I appreciate knowing there is that option.

Anyway, the point is I was a complete nervous wreck. My entire body functioned differently because of it. The heart palpitations, the nausea, the sweats, the sleeplessness, the nightmares. This was before any cancer treating drugs were put into my body. This was my brain doing flip flops. Some people had asked me if I had access to medical marijuana. I did not. A friend one day told me of a source and I can in fact acquire it legally here in California. Finally I saw a doctor (with an "MD." on his business card, anyway) who quite seriously looked over the details in my cancer folder and I was given my official letter that allows me to purchase it.

Not wanting to smoke, I had learned about the edible (chocolate) products that are offered. I learned through a friend it is very potent, so not to try too much. The first couple of times were pretty much off the charts. I didn't like it. I figured out how little I needed to benefit. It helped me eat which became a struggle mostly because I was nauseous from anxiety. I was terrified that I would become dangerously underweight and wither away.

By the time I went in for the port surgery and had been through two months of I-have-cancer anxiety, I weighed eighty-eight pounds. It was not the look I was going for and I did not want to lose another pound.

I don't sit around all day in a room filled with pot smoke wearing a bandana while playing guitar. The benefit of being able to tolerate and enjoy food helped my ability to stay strong and healthy and feel less anxious.

In the two years since I began working on this book, marijuana laws have shifted as states in the US de-criminalize and even legalize its use. I don't think people should walk (or drive) around stoned. But I'm glad medical use is legal here in California. I am an excellent example of its benefits. I know many who would agree. It still feels like a criminal act though, which is a shame considering the plethora of legal prescription drugs we're led to believe are safe, but often lead to overdose or addiction.

I'm happy to report I've gained some weight and I've made improvements to my diet like high protein and less sugar.

Listen, in my parallel universe I'm five foot seven and always wear flats. People can't even find me sometimes. I'll be walking along with my tall husband and he looks to his left, I'm not there. He looks to his right, and there I was the whole time. Airports are the worst. But I digress.

Home after Port Removal

Yesterday I had the port removed and the plastic surgeon created a new nipple (a typical day in the life of a breast cancer survivor I guess). I haven't seen it yet. It is covered in gauze and tape. I also had the belly button fixed as it stuck out too much from the previous surgery, and each end of the abdominal incision was corrected so that the little ends don't point out from the skin, which is (strangely) referred to as "dog ears". There is very little feeling on the breast so thankfully the nipple does not hurt. The port area feels rather raw. Other incisions are also sensitive but tolerable. I took pain medicine twice today and rested as it makes me sleepy.

People think that having gone through surgery before makes it less stressful. As the nurse so kindly pointed out, this is not the case. (Much to my surprise the nurse showed me her own port scar; she too is a survivor!) I still had to completely undress, remove my jewelry, put on the little blue hat and booties, get stuck in the arm with an IV and wait to be sedated. I hate the moment before sedation. I hate knowing that chemicals are being put in my body (yes, even after chemo) and I will have no control. Then of course I drift off and all is forgotten. Before I was given the "happy juice" my plastic surgeon came in and gently marked me in purple ink on each area. I felt in such good hands the whole time.

I woke in recovery with tears rolling down the sides of my face. My eyes were not yet open. I heard a nurse ask "Honey, are you having pain?" I was relieved to hear her voice. No. No pain. I was having a dream carried over from the previous night. Late into the night before the surgery as I drifted off to sleep I cried tears of joy (mixed in with some pre-surgery anxiety) that I was finally having the port removed. Finally no tube protruding from my skin near my collar bone. Finally no big button through my thin upper chest. Finally the end of the reason I needed the port in the first place. It has been almost one year.

Goodbye port. I won't miss you. Thanks for everything.

Today is Valentine's Day

Exactly one year ago tomorrow I began my first chemotherapy treatment. Is this the end of this journey? Is today the day that I am done?

I have landed on my feet. I have weathered the storm. I have braved the open sea. I have become even more, forever, me.

Fortitude

Happiness is neither virtue nor pleasure nor this thing nor that,
but simply growth.
We are happy when we are growing.
William Butler Yeats

Thanks Christina Aguilera

Almost every morning while I am trying to fix this impossible short hair and putting on my make-up I listen to the song "Fighter" by Christina Aguilera. The chorus really nails it.

The Feeling That Doesn't Go Away

The overwhelming feeling that goes in and out of my conscious thought is the fear that I am totally undesirable now. That I am ruined and have lost my membership in the looking-pretty-good-most-of-the-time category. Even though no one can see my scars, except for my husband, I know they are there. And my short hair doesn't do me any favors. It's that stupid post chemo hair that puffs out. I'm not complaining. I'm glad to have hair of course. I'm glad to be alive of course. I'm glad I can get up every day and think, and do and be. *Obviously*. But there is the terrible sadness I must fight every day.

I think it is mixed in with some chemo fog. I constantly write myself notes so I won't forget the simplest things. I've always been a list maker. At the end of each day I write on post-it notes and stick them on my computer (old school style) so I'll see them first thing in the morning. First I have to remember to write the note!

Current List of Paranoia

Sugar (except for dark chocolate which is supposed to be beneficial)
Pasta
Alcohol
Restaurant food
Exhaust fumes
Walking by someone smoking a cigarette
My right breast
Neck lymph nodes
Stress
Blaming myself for cancer
Pressuring myself to do too much
Coming off weird since I'm obviously in the cancer bubble
Anything perfumed
A child coughing

What I Am Capable of Doing about it

Make best food choices possible
Meditate away from stress
Keep regular doctor appointments
Find the things that I truly love and embrace those things
Let others take care of things I don't have time to do
In moments of anger or frustration, find a happy image and breathe
Walk
Find a positive outlet for my nervous energy
Stop feeling guilty for needing ME time
If I am happy, my family will be happy
Keep going to therapy
Dance
Read
Sing

It does take a long time to feel "normal" whatever that is.

The weather is lovely today. I pruned the lavender and cut back the purple grass. I love getting messy and digging out the old, dying leaves. I feel energized by nurturing new growth. I feel alive in the garden. Being surrounded by nature even in the smallest way is a great way to get outside of the sadness, at least for a little while.

What Was This All For?

Afraid of dying, afraid of living. That's no way to live.

Being a Mom

I wasn't a very good mom last year. No one would blame me. I was buried in cancer stuff. It was rough. I slept. I watched lots of movies. I needed my own space. I still sleep in late. I toss and turn at night because of "chemopause" hot flashes and have become selfish about rest. My kids are just going to have to understand. My daughter wanted a ride to school this morning but I was not ready (and Chuck was already gone). It's walking distance but she was upset. I can't cater to it every time. I feel badly but I'm trying to focus my energy as best I can on the things that need attention. I feel I need to keep reminding myself to put *me* first. It's slightly refreshing.

As a mother I've put some things ahead of my own personal development. Then I was kicked in the ass and knocked down. A curve ball. A new road. A different path. Life is full of twists and turns. Every so often you have to look at your priorities and figure out what's best.

Focus

Focus positive energy. Breathe out negative energy. Must focus on goals at hand. Must try not to get distracted by nonsense. Do away with non-productive thinking. Focus on happy. Focus on sound. Focus on good energy. Must do this. With all my might. With every waking moment must focus. Rest and focus. Everything will fall into place.

Thanks chemo brain. Glad we cleared that up.

Repeat this often. Don't forget!!

It's the Tiny Things That Really Matter

Yippee for eyelashes!

Being Alive

I wake up in the morning and have to remind myself that every-thing is okay now. That I am not in a current state of trauma. That whatever happens in the future is out of my hands for the moment. Sometimes I don't want to get out of bed; it is so hard to begin another day of worry or fear. But then I remember I was given a fake breast, my abdominal scar has healed very well, my port scar continues to heal and I have more energy now. I have to remind myself that today I can live. I can make good choices about the foods I eat and the way I take in the day. I can pause and rest and hydrate when I need to. I can follow my instincts but slow down when necessary. The anxiousness does tend to linger long after the body has healed.

When I was first diagnosed I thought it would be a six-month journey. Then I realized it was a year. Now I realize it's even more than that. Wishing it hadn't happened isn't productive. The hours in the day occur one way or the other.

Might as well brush my teeth and get on with it.

I'm Getting the Hang of This

New response if someone asks me how I'm feeling: "Feeling like crap, but I get up every morning anyway"

Not Just My Fight Anymore

I am not trying to obsess over the past. I am not trying to stay stuck in a place of pain or pity. But I cannot un-know what I know now. I do not take comfort that I was treated and can now walk away going back to my ordinary life. It is bigger than me, this thing I have gone through. Mostly it is heartache knowing that right now a woman is being told she has breast cancer. I refuse to accept this. I need to tell of my experience. It is ludicrous that millions of women go through this.

Can I Have My Boring, Straight Hair Back, Please?

Do I seem obsessed with it all? The hair, the recovery, the process? Maybe I am.

Working with chemo hair presents some challenges. I'm delighted to have hair of course. But it is very strange, poofy hair.

Some suggestions:

Condition your new hair more than you think you should. The more moisture, the more shiny and less poofy.

Use Moroccan oil. It adds shine.

I don't recommend permanent hair color but if you decide to do it wait until at least six months of new hair. Have stray hair on the neck trimmed by a professional.

Try out different styles as it grows; push it back, bring it forward, etc. You have to play around with this new hair until it does something decent.

This is Not the Time to Quit Being Me

Many of us support group girls are trying to get back to "normal". I hate to break it to you but normal has changed. There is nothing like a bout with a life-threatening disease to put things in perspective and cut out a lot of nonsense. My post-cancer new normal feels every moment with such vibration and possibility I feel like I'm going to burst.

It's good to have energy again. I am enjoying being alive in between forcing myself to *not* think about cancer. Recently I've felt angry about the whole thing and even thought the anger might help facilitate this story. But the truth is I don't want to live in anger. It helped for a long time. It absolutely gave me strength when I needed it.

I am learning to accept that some things that happen are not fair. It's a hard lesson. I can't hold on tight forever. Someone could have told me this from the start but I had to learn it for myself. I've had to let go in my own way. I'm learning to let go of trying to fix it all, or understand it all.

It is a time for healing, a little selfishness (or a lot) and plenty of celebration.

I keep wondering when I will write the last journal entry. Thinking about it must mean that soon I will be ready to move forward one more step toward the rest of my life and further away from what was. It couldn't be happening at a more perfect time, the very beginning of spring.

The birds are chirping, the flowers are blooming and so am I.

Less Pity

Feeling less sorry for myself these days. More ready to look in the mirror and see what I see.

Watched a French film the other day called "Rust and Bone". In the movie a woman who works at a marine park in France has a freak accident when one of the massive dolphins rushes toward the platform, injuring the people directing the dolphins in the show. The woman wakes up in the hospital and in a haze realizes both of her legs are gone from the knees down. She goes through extraordinary sadness of course. She even wants to die. The movie shows her long process toward living again in a new way, forever changed from her experience.

Anyone who has gone through not only something tragic but also something physically traumatic must take time to grieve. There is no escaping the despair. But there is life after such difficulty.

Taking Flight from the House of Cancer

The check-in area at the oncology office is filled with people quietly waiting for their destiny. You sign in, go sit down, and wait for your name to be called. As patients come in and out you wonder what ailment they have and what story they have to tell. Once in a while a bald woman walks in. Or an older man arrives accompanied by his daughter. Or you spot a young couple sitting in the shadows and it's hard to tell which one is the patient because they both look calm and lovely.

The nurse comes out and checks her list. She calls a name but it is not yours. You wait. You anticipate being taken to the next area where you will be weighed and your blood will be drawn.

It is all very civilized in the realm of what is at best, difficult.

Every single person on that staff, every doctor, anyone with a name tag who passes through, is there to help save your life.

There are many patients ahead of you and unfortunately many more to come after you've gone home. You realize there is an entire community of sick people waiting to get better. You calculate as you sit there how your life will look when this part is behind you.

Your glimpse of the future is the woman who has clearly grown her hair back to a chic, intentional style, standing at the front desk speaking to the kind-faced attendant. You look for the signs of "better" all around you and know that when you have gone through the series of treatments prescribed for you, when you have been given the drugs developed for the thing that went wrong with you, you will visit this place less often. You will calendar in fewer and fewer follow-ups until your time is your own again.

The doctors here take in the unlucky broken birds allowing them to return as safely as possible to their nests.

The quiet waiting is your safe space to envision your future once your wing is repaired. You will fly once again, possibly even better than before. You will fly to new places, new heights, looking back, yes, but keeping forward motion, staying strong, facing the wind.

Wherever I Go

I enter the hotel elevator as an imposter. I traveled here in the past, the *other* me, the *before* me, the *non-cancer* me, the *unknowing* me. This time I am a different guest. There is no escaping the truth. All the way across the country I still have a scar from hip to hip, a fake breast with scars on it, evidence of the port, and of course the short hair. No matter where I am this is the result. Not that I expected to feel different or relieved of my reality. No, as I bathe after a wonderful day seeing the sights of Washington DC, I come back to what has transpired. Never before have I slept in a hotel feeling my replacement breast against the unfamiliar hotel sheets. I observe my new reflection in the mirror above the counter that holds the miniature coffee machine next to the little blow dryer attached to the wall.

It is all new, all a gift, all a reward of the hard work. A new "me" enters into every situation, at every turn, at every opportunity. I am so grateful to get to see my little niece for the first time, so very grateful to see the cherry blossoms, to see the White House, to enjoy the care of the hotel environment, to have that awful hotel coffee. It is all perfect in what is completely imperfect.

Flying Home

Many years after 9-11, I feared airplanes. My stomach would be in knots on take-off and landing. I would have anxiety for hours, even days before each flight. Cancer knocked all of that aside. Fear of flying is no match for a disgusting group of misguided cells. Gee, thanks cancer. I can walk through just about whatever comes my way.

I fear my own feelings less. Bring on the day. I have nothing to lose.

The List Continues

I carry around with me the paranoia of exposing myself to any environment. It seems that at every turn, there is danger. Exhaust fumes from cars and buses is my biggest fear of late. Here are some others that cause me angst on a daily basis:

Anything fried
Sugar

Any processed food
Someone coughing or sneezing in public
Public bathrooms
Ingredients in make-up
Cheese
Alcohol (apparently studies show it increases cancer risk)

Why, you ask? Because any one of these things has either germs or chemicals, or potentially bad hormones. I wish I knew exactly what caused my cancer. It would be nice to be at ease with my surroundings. Even if I ingest only the most natural foods, walking across the street while breathing is a risk. It's maddening. The anxiety runs through me in waves.

And:

Cigarette smoke of course. One of the worst of all.

Hair

I look at women with beautiful silky hair and want to weep. It is a longing that gets stuck in my throat. It doesn't matter that I've received compliments on my short do. It's not even that I hate it. I want normal hair again. This new curly chemo hair is a constant reminder of what happened.

I miss my old eyelashes.

When

It's been almost one year from the date that I finished chemotherapy. It's hard to believe. When do I stop talking about it? When do I stop publicly acknowledging what I've been through as though it is still in the present? When do I stop attributing the ripple effect of everything that occurred? When is my life not emotionally caught up in the fact that I had a life-threatening disease and lost a body part because of it? When do I talk about normal, everyday things and not reflect on how it correlates to my breast cancer experience? When do I stop using the cancer card? Am I using it as a crutch? Do I feel sorry for myself? Shouldn't I? When do I stop feeling angry, alienated, ugly, afraid? When do I put the past behind me?

Do I get to use the emotional energy toward new and exciting things? What do I do when I have that sinking feeling, remembering my vulnerability? How do I make that positive leap from fear to courage? Why can't it be right now. Today. Here.

Jealous (again)

I'm jealous of people who have furthered their goals while I had to spend the last twelve months regaining my health. The bliss of ignorance is a thing of the past.

No More an Alien

She is human again. She is sleeping fairly well. She feels pretty much like she did before. But then she looks in the mirror. Staring back at her is an older lady with a short haircut. Her face has changed. When she sees her image in a photograph there appears a different expression. Her cheeks look fuller. Her eyebrows are not what she remembers.

People ask her how she feels. She says "great". She never felt sick anyway until the chemo regimen began. She never knew she had a time bomb inside of her.

But now she doesn't.

The Party

I select what to wear looking forward to the gathering of family and friends and anticipate the familiar questions and comments; "how are you feeling?", "are you ok?", and maybe even, "you look great".

Out my front door I go, a nice version of the self I envision, feeling good about my clothes, hair and make-up. Understated elegance with a modern twist is usually the goal.

The party is held at a generously sized family home, traditionally furnished. Floral prints adorn the walls. Guests mingle and migrate toward the backyard where drinks are being served. The evening is a perfect expression of smiling faces, easy conversation, and birthday wishes for the host.

When I arrive within "hello" distance of the crowd I am welcomed by the gentle eyes of those few who know what happened, hugging me a little longer than usual, simply wanting me to be well. I feel a pang of anxiety as I allow the curiosity, the recognition, of what they know I had to endure. I receive compliments on my chic, short hair but all the same wish I had silky straight locks like before.

It is refreshing to enjoy the company of nice people as though I am like any other normal human being. My husband is a terrific conversationalist and knows something about everything. He tends to universally put people at ease with his ability to find a relatable subject. We wind up talking to a couple about where we each live and where we grew up. We talk about our kids and our families, college, and cars. A woman briefly explains that she is caring for her mother who has cancer and only nine months to live. A moment of reflection and concern is felt as we stand under the stars each cradling special birthday drinks from the bar.

Live music floats through the air and the woman who shared her story about her ailing mother asks me what I do. This past year I would usually just say that I am an interior designer. This time I decide to also include that I am coming back from the difficult year that it was. The truth is the woman had unknow-ingly offered a safe bridge for me to cross. Had she not mentioned her dying mother I probably would not have disclosed to this person who I'd only just met, the two-sentence version of my very recent time with cancer. Since she had shared her difficulty I felt permission to share mine. As a new card carrying member of the Cancer Club I cannot deny that my work and life have been obviously, temporarily, thrown off course.

I am surprised at how little it stings, revealing I had recently had cancer. I still hate the word and wish it didn't exist at all, for anyone, anywhere, ever. But it is difficult to obscure the attention it commands even long after the emergency is over. It so happens that last year at this time I was going to treatment every three weeks. Last year was, without hesitation, the most brutal time of my life. It just so happens that this is still my truth.

The rest of the evening is sprinkled with fine food, intriguing anecdotes and much laughter. It is easy to enjoy.

The long road I traveled, now finding myself at this party, took me through pitch darkness and completely unfamiliar places. I had no choice but to ask for help back to safety and something feels different now, emotionally, physically. Perhaps it is the calm spring air or the beautiful home. Perhaps it is feeling just right in what I chose to wear or the happy demeanor of the hosts. Or it is all of these things plus the advantage of time. On this glorious night of food, love, friendship, and celebration, it is clear; I am that much farther away from what was and that much closer to what can be. Although it wasn't so long ago and the questions and comments about my well-being continue to require my attention, I am no longer in the throes of being a breast cancer patient.

It is finally true after all. I am, on this very day, right now, unbelievably, thankfully, gratefully, at *this* moment in time, a cancer survivor. Forever scarred on the surface of my skin, forever, I am one of those women home from battle, strong, afraid, but alive.

Perhaps as I keep healing, the need to tell will fade. There is no sense hiding it away though; this dark note in the music of my life. It will always be. It is there, heard more easily when all else has gone quiet. It is in my step, and on my lips. But the lyrics to my song continue and I'll dance as long as I can. Yes, I guess that's what I'll do.

The Yoga Class

I value a good stretch like anyone else. This was my second class, and probably my third time doing yoga and I felt enthusiastic about getting started. The previous class was taught by a substitute. I liked her. She was direct and pleasant. This instructor, who I hadn't met but teaches the class regularly, seemed to take pride in connecting with the students in a very personal way. She knew the ailments of each person and firmly directed our arms or legs to the right or left whenever needed. I'm not bad for someone starting out. I'm pretty limber but my bones did ache under the pressure of unfamiliar twists and turns.

This was the first time the instructor had seen me and at the start of class asked if I had signed in at the front desk. I said yes. She asked again, "You have the pink card?" I told her that I had previously enrolled and came to class the day of the substitute. Then I realized the instructor thought I didn't belong. It was a class for cancer survivors. Finally, I said, pointing to my hair, "Can't you tell?" Of course my hair doesn't look like new post-chemo hair to most people but I know what I looked like before, with straight hair down to my shoulders.

The woman to my right looked at me and said "But you're so young". I told her I'm not as young as she thinks. Then I looked around at the other women in the room, only five of us, and I said, "None of you look like you had cancer either". We all smiled, understanding that you can't always tell when someone has had cancer. We got into a brief discussion about how it can strike at any age and it's not our fault. The instructor was also a cancer survivor and she offered her words of wisdom as we sat with our legs crossed, facing the mirror.

The cool down at the end of class lasted way too long. Did she notice my eyes were open the whole time? Did she see me trying to get something out of my eye? Was I breathing wrong? I wanted to get up and run out of the room. At the end of class she looked at me and said, "You need to learn how to relax". Who is this yoga instructor to tell me to relax? Don't you know I have a lot of catching up to do? Don't you know I spent months and months healing? Don't you know I'm trying to get on with it? Haven't you read my blog, about how I have lots of energy now?

Sure, I know, I need to relax, get out of my head and be present. Maybe I'm bursting with renewed vigor. Did you ever think of *that*, nice yoga lady?

Okay, maybe I do need to relax. That is why I'm taking a yoga class, right? Telling someone to relax is like telling someone to not be hungry.

I'll see how the class goes next time. I'll give it a chance.

Maybe I shouldn't have had that second cup of coffee.

Maybe brisk walking is more my cup of tea.

I later learned that the "cool down" is *Shavasana*, or death pose. Clearly I have worked very hard to *not* do the *death pose*, thank you! No wonder it felt so very wrong. I appreciate the value of meditation but I am too busy jumping for joy!

Pelvic Ultrasound (Thanks to Tamoxifen Risks)

Scheduled for two weeks from now. Nervous. What else can I be?

Please

Please God don't let my body fail again. I don't think I could do this more than once. Please God I'll do my best. I want to live until I'm too old, until I'm ready to go, until I can slip away peacefully. I face this thought and want to push it down and that's what is so hard each day.

But I will eat cookies from time to time. And I will drink wine from time to time. I might have white bread or candy. Not much. But I will. And I will occasionally eat meat. My diet is excellent most of the time; salads, fruit, organic chicken, no soda at all, salmon, not much milk (just cream in my coffee). I swear I'll do what I can. I will take vitamin D with calcium as instructed. Just don't destroy me with breast cancer. Please.

Thanks God. I appreciate it.

Last May

I missed spring last year. My second to last chemo was mother's day weekend and I slept through it. I missed the celebration of flowers and moms. This year I feel acutely aware of so much beauty, blue sky, bright flowers, gentle breezes. It's all new again. I missed my favorite season last year. It's not that I was unaware. But under the duress of treatment everything shifts temporarily. This year I am truly alive.

Another Message to the Temple Board of Directors

My co-president term had ended but I was still a member of the board. I began to realize I had missed many months of meetings during my recovery and I felt less than equipped to contribute to the issues at hand. Not only that, being a board member means being privy to behind the scenes stress and frankly, I did not want it hanging over me. It was time to put *me* first.

Dear Wonderful Members of the Board,
First, I'd like to say congrats on a year of hard work and dedication.

You may or may not know I am stepping down from the board at the end of July. I certainly did miss a lot of activity this past year but I am grateful to have had the opportunity to serve with you.

While I can't honestly say I'll miss the hard work and challenges that come with being a board member, I will miss the camaraderie and sense of contribution I have been so fortunate to be a part of for many years.

It is hard to step away, but my focus continues to be long-term health and to de-stress whenever possible. When I'm ready, I know there are many wonderful opportunities for involvement at our temple and I am grateful for that.

I wish you all the very best in the new term and thank you again for your kindness over the past year and a half. Much of it is a blur but I've always felt comforted and so very blessed by our special community.

With love and admiration,
Alicia

Observations

Breasts Do Not a Woman Make

A woman becoming transgender has her breasts removed. She doesn't want them. They are meaningless to her. Rather, what they mean to her she does not like. She has a sweet, soft voice, a beautiful smile, a delicate face with good cheekbones and white teeth. Dark skin, she is from an exotic place. But she does not want to be a she. She has removed her breasts.

My new left breast is a security blanket. I could live without my breasts if I had to. Of course I could. I'd be sad. I'd feel incomplete. But I could do it. She feels more genuine without them. My breasts no longer match exactly but after the areola tattoo they'll be okay.

She chose to have her breasts cut away. I could never have imagined doing such a thing had it not been for cancer. Modern medicine sure has some tricks up its sleeve.

The $60,000 Boob

Two of my favorite T.V. shows growing up were: *The Six Million Dollar Man,* and of course, *The Bionic Woman.* Well now I have a $60,000 dollar boob. In total, saving my life came to somewhere around $300,000 for all of the chemo, steroid shots, doctor visits, hospital stays, etc., not including expenses for hats, anxiety medications, therapy sessions, vitamins, and high quality protein powders. Had it not been for medical insurance through my husband's job with a company that supports employees worldwide I don't know what we would have done.

My husband's employer essentially saved my life and bought me a boob. Each holiday season they have a lovely party. We got some nice pictures two months before I would lose all of my hair.

We've still had many co-pays but nothing compared to what it could have been. Without insurance sometimes you can't even get an appointment with a doctor. What the hell would I have done?

Maybe I would have gone through treatment and then had the mastectomy without reconstruction. That means I'd be sitting here right now with one breast.

The changes to my body have been a difficult adjustment. But this is the price of modern medicine as we know it.

To have the lingering anxiety of finances on top of being diagnosed with a deadly disease is unacceptable and I'm excited to start fundraising for the Avon Walk. The ridiculous thing is, it could be said we are creating our own toxic environment for which we then pay the price when we get a disease and all we've got so far is to treat it with toxic concoctions. It's a vicious cycle and I find it to be a very sad state of affairs.

I'm grateful for my $60,000 dollar boob. She's pretty spectacular. She'll do just fine.

Hopefully the Affordable Care Act initiated this year will be an important first step to help all women and men have access to healthcare.

Scared All Over Again

Like a child, afraid. Going for an MRI today. Took a little Xanax to relieve the physical sensation. The energy is sucked out of me trying to hold in and be brave. Intellectually I am fairly sure everything will be fine. But it is the process of being exposed, being stuck in the arm with the needle which injects the dye into my veins, which I will taste in my mouth. It is holding still during the procedure, barely breathing. I had forgotten how scary and unfamiliar the MRI space is. It used to make sure all of the cancer was gone. Now it is to make sure it hasn't come back.

I feel uneasy, queasy, outside of myself. Must be good to

myself today, not try too hard to pressure myself. Need mental energy to get through it even though it is a fairly easy procedure compared to some others. Still, it is the space it takes up in my brain; planning the time to get there, undressing from the waist up, lying down on the cold, hard plastic, electronically guided into the small space as the technician leaves the room to enter her glass box and start.

I had forgotten. I am being forced to remember. Forced to check my body. Forced to include this into my day, to make sure, to say, yes, I'm still okay.

Forward Motion

The more I think about it, the more I realize participating in the Avon Walk is the end point to this story. What a nice way to bring purpose and celebration to it all.

The "M" Word

I didn't utter the "M" word to my fifteen-year-old daughter until two days ago. Last year I wasn't ready to tell her that my entire breast was going to be removed. She was fourteen when I found out I was going to have the surgery. She was blossoming into a beautiful young woman and I didn't have it in me to say out loud to her what was to be my reality. Of course my daughter and son knew I was having surgery but I omitted the word "mastectomy" from my conversations with them. The word probably did float out of other people's mouths from time to time, but not mine. I told them the truth; that the previous surgery; the lumpectomy, did not remove enough tissue and more needed to be removed and would then be reconstructed which is why the second surgery would take a long time; as it turned out, a whopping twelve hours.

As the days revealed more of what was to be the course of my treatment I doled out information in small, manageable bits. In one conversation right after I was diagnosed, my sweet and rather shy daughter looked at me and asked "Could it happen to me too?" I had no road map in my hand to answer this question. No one had told me what questions to expect from my children. No one told me how to address them. (I eventually came across a helpful article in a UCLA publication during my second chemotherapy treatment.)

I could dance around the word mastectomy for a while but I couldn't bullshit around the fact that there are no guarantees in life. I answered as honestly as I could and told my daughter "It is unlikely that it will. As long as you are aware of your body and get health checks, in the years to come as you grow up medical advances will be even better than they are now and you'll take care of whatever needs taking care of". It pained me to not be able to produce more promise, but I hoped that my honest approach would satisfy what she needed to know. Fortunately I was negative for the BRCA gene, which has helped her (and me) feel more assured. But if the test *had* revealed something, we would have figured out our next steps. Although, to think that my lovely daughter would ever face what I went through causes my throat to close up and my ribs to feel as though they are caving in.

Initially I was more caught up in protecting my kids from my fear of losing my hair than I was of losing my breast. I knew right from the start I was going to follow traditional methods of treatment despite the frightening levels of toxicity. My daughter had become familiar with the character on Desperate Housewives, Lynette Scavo played by Felcity Huffman, and this seemed to help her grapple with my situation, and we would talk about the character from time to time. (You never know where opportunities for discussion will crop up.)

My then sixteen-year-old son had not seen my bald head. I had asked him one day if he wanted to see what I looked like. I was getting used to it, and truth be told I was tired of walking around the house constantly covering up, but he firmly said "No", and I respected his feelings. Perhaps being a boy it was even harder for him to comprehend and at the same time he didn't want to know. Not long after I proposed to show him my baldness he ultimately did catch a glimpse of my peach fuzz and it was a non-event. I told both kids that even though I would look worse for a while I was getting better. I needed to hear myself say that out loud.

After the breast reconstruction it took about four weeks for me to stand up completely straight. Again, I told my kids I wouldn't be like that forever and eventually would be standing up again. As I continuously reassured them I was reassuring myself. I felt good about my decision to reconstruct but it was not made easily.

The other day with my daughter in the car, we somehow got to talking about breast cancer. Maybe I said something about how excited I was for the upcoming Avon walk in Santa Barbara. Maybe she said something about her friend at school who had lost her hair during treatment this past school year. In any case, I finally said "Yes, I had a mastectomy on the left breast and they reconstructed it in the same surgery", and clarifying that "no, I didn't have an implant", to her questioning the timeline of what I had done.

Finally it was made clear to her what had happened. I hoped that finally she could see I was alright after all. Finally I didn't hide from the "M" word. Maybe the whole subject is on our radar now and we're more comfortable with it. News like actress Angelina Jolie's procedure brought it to light recently which probably helped my ability to speak the truth. Although the results of the surgery were pretty spectacular I felt so devastated over the changes forced on my body that before that moment in the car I couldn't bring myself to give her all of the details; at least not all at once. Not only has she matured before my eyes but the depth of my own despair lingered.

I never had all that much regard for my breasts in the first place. But losing one made me confront them, appreciate them, and mourn the loss. It may be that I needed to protect myself from the cold hard facts of what I was going through more than my daughter needed protection, but we are in a better frame of mind now to look back and gain perspective. I hope she doesn't feel as though I withheld information in a deceitful way. That was not the intention but now I can see she may wonder why it took me so long to just say what was happening. She's grown emotionally in the past year and a half and that too has helped encourage the level of conversation.

I would like to be able to say that I was the last person in line for a mastectomy. Sadly I cannot. I wish with all my heart that one day someone will be the very last patient requiring such a procedure and that detection becomes eradication. That one day there will not be such a discussion between a mother and her children and we can be rid of *all* cancer.

Facing sudden illness, or in the case of cancer, the slow process of living in the unknown is difficult to navigate. Families each have a unique dynamic which plays a role in how we express ourselves to each other. In the case of having two teenage children I felt the strain of their wanting and being capable of understanding but my reluctance to force the frightening, ugly truth upon them.

More than ever before (not surprisingly) I live each day enormously grateful for another sunrise. Any time I feel off course I put myself back into a place of gratitude. The little annoyances of daily life are no match for the upheaval our family faced last year. My husband and I have become closer. It might even be true that my kids appreciate me a little bit more than they did before I was diagnosed. I'll take it. Hopefully they too have a sense of gratitude in their lives. Maybe they now know how much I wanted to protect them. Maybe they now know that at least for today it's gonna be alright and that's all any of us can know. It doesn't get better than that. It's all icing on the cake from here.

On the Edge

As I was imagining my death I was never more alive. Now that I have settled down I feel less compulsion to write. How tragic.

The Fog

I still get foggy, unfocused, muddled. I write about it because I know it is a different me and a remnant of what my body went through. I know this but it is frustrating to feel like an outsider from my own brain. I continuously need to pull myself back from some strange abyss. Some place where words slow down, emotions become strained. I know "chemopause" explains some of it. It seems to me that the hot flashes affect my brain. Sometimes I give in and stop to meditate. Sometimes I decide to nourish with crunchy raw vegetables. Sometimes, like now I stop to write it down; this strange feeling that comes over me that I never used to feel.

I'll leave it up to the professionals to continue documenting how chemotherapy and other drugs affect cognitive function. I'm here to report that it does. Period.

Celebration

How Do I Say Thank You?

To Oncologist Dr. Sara Hurvitz. Thank you for saving my life.

To Nurse Kim for the hugs.

To the nurses who administered six chemo treatments plus eleven Herceptin.

To the nurse who gave me a Neulasta shot the day after each chemo and massaged my arm afterward.

To the surgeon who implanted the port in my chest, and the anesthesiologist who understood how afraid I was and checked on me throughout the procedure.

To the scheduling guy who is a fellow Scorpio and made me laugh the day he tried on my wig (on his chocolate-brown bald head).

To Dr. Ryan who told me the news and calmly witnessed my rage and confusion.

To the UCLA radiology department who found the two lumps in a mammogram and gave me the heads-up warning of concern, and for the gentle treatment during the MRIs and biopsies.

To surgeon Dr. Nova Foster who produced the most invisible lymph node incision, and who was willing to try the lumpectomy, but ultimately removed my left breast.

To Dr. Charles Tseng, the most gentle, kind, and brilliant plastic surgeon ever to walk the face of the earth.

To the nurses during my four-day stay in the hospital after the reconstruction, who helped me get up out of the bed when I could barely move.

To the medical tattoo artist Laura Albano for the amazing areola tattoo.

To Nurse Gilbert, who administered my first chemo, and didn't get nervous when we realized the dose of Benadryl was causing me a problem.

To Kauser Ahmed, who led the UCLA support group, always with extraordinary patience and wisdom.

To the support group girls, Arlene, Carol, Jill, Lois, and Phyllis, who faced the hurdles alongside me while they were going through it too, and lifted me up when I didn't know I could do it. To their partners who met each other and felt that deep connection only caregivers could understand.

To Susan and Jim for the brilliant gift of a full year of house cleaning.

To Amy, owner of Created Hair for the amazing human hair wig.

To my mother, Susan, who remained calm, provided plenty of laughs, and told me how proud she was of how I handled it all.

To my stepdad, Henry, who helped me stay strong by listening, and talking about his heart surgery from years before, reminding me how amazing the human spirit is.

To my dad's wife Jo-Ann, who called every week and spoke so kindly, listened to my nervous chatter, and for sending the Carol Burnett DVD collection.

To my dad, Steve, who flew out from New Jersey numerous times (in the midst of his own medical issues), hugged me tight, and took a fantastic photo of me in my state of baldness after chemo number four.

To my husband, Charles, who held me as I sobbed more deeply than I ever knew possible, who stayed incredibly strong and was a voice of reason when I thought I was going insane, who drove me to a distant project meeting because I had an emotional breakdown that morning for no good reason whatsoever.

To my two beautiful, extraordinary miracles, Rachel and Bradley, for being the very reason I need to be here, for being able to laugh again, for being the kind, considerate people we need in the world.

To Rabbi Neil who contacted me on the phone numerous

times offering comfort by simply listening.

To Roselee, for her strength and kindness, with a twist of sassiness.

To my sister Carlie who rallied support from afar, connecting my local friends together who brought meals to my doorstep after the big surgery, and for the care package of herbal tinctures and the beautiful purple stone necklace.

To my friends Etty, Hanna, Sheri and Wendy who were there during various times with nourishment, a friendly ear, and a trip to the salon for the shave.

To cousin Minda, a voice of reason and a good measure of much needed humor.

To my sister Nole, who had excellent timing and gave birth to her beautiful child, bringing sunshine into our families lives.

To my brother Chad, who texted hellos and how are yous often.

To my sister Elys, for reading my posts and sending messages of love.

To aunt Nora who told me it would be a blip, which was in fact comforting to hear.

To my mother-in-law, Mary, who sent the most gorgeous flowers and gave me one of her orchid paintings knowing it would cheer me up.

To many, many more people who gave me random hugs, sent flowers, cards, emails, called, and helped me know that with their love I would get through it.

To Laurel who urged that I post "Time" on Huffington Post which encouraged me to share my writing for the first time in my life, and led to a book deal and home decor web articles.

To Dr. Dennis Slamen, whom I have never met, who developed Herceptin which is one of the most important drugs I was given.

To my little poodle Skipper for cuddling with me when I was bald, tired, emotional, scared, and pimple faced. I know he can't read but he was my little furry ball of comfort and cuteness, and it helped.

To a friend for referring me to the dispensary.

To the many women I've never met who bravely blogged about their experience offering a glimpse into their lives so that I could better understand mine as I searched the internet late into the night trying to make sense of the unimaginable.

Although I've mentioned so many, there are still many more. I am forever grateful for the words of encouragement and presence of so much love.

The Stories

UCLA Simms Mann Cocktail Party Fundraiser

I was asked by the psychologist who leads the support group if I'd be willing to speak at a fundraiser for the Simms Mann Center. Of course I said yes! I had been sharing some of my posts with her and although I never imagined it would lead me to this day, I'm glad it did. Here's what I said, in the company of board members, oncologists (including mine), past patients, and prospective donors.

When I was diagnosed with breast cancer and met with (my hero) Dr. Sara Hurvitz she assured me and my husband that treatment is better than ever before and that I would live. But I felt I needed support outside of my family circle. They didn't know all that much about breast cancer and with two teenagers at home, a hardworking and supportive husband, concerned family far and wide, I knew I needed a place to find my balance and not feel alone. I did reach out to friends and relatives who understood, or had been through it.

Many people lovingly reached out to me as well. I explored vitamin supplements, cancer-fighting foods, meditation, yoga, laughter, and whatever else was going to get me through. And yes, late at night I searched the internet way too much.

At my very first oncology appointment I was referred to the Simms Mann Center. It didn't take me long to get in my car and drive to Westwood. The emotions I felt were so intense I couldn't believe this was the experience for millions of women and millions of others who have experienced other types of cancer.

On my first visit to Simms Mann I was greeted by psychologist Kauser Ahmed who asked a few questions to be sure I was in the right place. In her office tears rolled down my face as I explained my diagnosis and my need to find a place to express how I felt without relying exclusively on my patient husband who had already held me tight many evenings as I cried in his arms. She assured me I was in the right place. I learned that there are a number of resources and I was welcome to try them out any time. I felt such relief that I could have a connection to these services without additional costs, to help me get well.

I went to support group regularly where I addressed my concerns for my children who were not always able to talk about their feelings. I also spoke with a clinical trainee at the center privately who provided insights on how I could deal with my feelings of guilt for feeling like a burden, and my teenage son's fear of expressing his feelings because he didn't want to burden me. Those insights gave me language I needed to talk to my son so that we could be a family team together. "Give your kids more credit for being able to help you", she had said; a revelation to me after feeling so protective of them. My learning process helped my husband, my daughter and my close family. When I told my parents I was attending a support group they were so thankful I had somewhere to turn. I know at times they felt helpless, struggling to figure out what would be most beneficial to me as I went through the rollercoaster ride of treatment and surgeries. Each week they would ask "did you go to support group?" and because they knew I had these resources they knew I was not alone.

The thing is, cancer is not just about cancer. The emotional impact reached every aspect of my life. The Simms Mann support helped me face issues unique to me while I was in the midst of fighting the fight.

In group I met women who were getting through the most difficult days. They were achieving what I could not imagine and moving forward. It was encouraging to meet these women in person and know that they were real people experiencing the same fears and thoughts as me. The group was my lifeline for about a year. It takes time, more time than I could have known, to regain physical and emotional strength. That group was my safe place to feel uneasy, to wrestle with dark thoughts, to share tips and information, and to cheer each other on as we reached treatment milestones. I met women who seemed so brave and yet I found it hard to see myself that way. The support I received in that room helped me gain confidence in myself, and better prepared me for the future living with my new reality.

I would be a different person today had I not had the benefit of the group and all that Simms Mann offers. I would have been alone in my thoughts, overwhelmed with fear, confusion and unresolved anxiety.

The women I met will be forever in my mind. We love each other. We continue to support each other even if it has nothing to do with our breasts. Although it is true that any time we're in a room together we eventually lift up our shirts, compare how we've healed and how our experience has affected our lives. The group was my ray of sunshine. For a period of time, it was the only place I wanted to be, to let it out, to find my new normal.

I will be forever grateful to those women and to the Simms Mann Center for holding me up, for treating me with such kindness, for allowing me to express my feelings, shed my tears, and find strength by drawing upon the experience of other women who understood me completely.

I am honored to be here with you tonight to express my gratitude and hopefully give you a sense of my experience. I know that the women I remain close with are all grateful for each other and for the Simms Mann support, one of the many unexpected gifts of my cancer journey.

Thank you.

My Stage Debut at a Spoken Word Salon in Los Angeles

My friend Wendy Hammers, actress, producer and writer, runs a writing workshop and a story salon called *Tasty Words* ™. Once I started posting some of my essays on line I continued to honor the writer in me and began attending her workshop. Wendy and I met about fourteen years ago (my, how time flies) when our boys were three years old in nursery school. Through the years, we'd call on each other regularly for play dates, sleepovers, pick-ups, drop-offs, stuff like that. We've shared our mommy angst together and have had plenty of great times with and without our kids.

By the time I began Wendy's workshop I had already begun putting together this book. Her support and safe space for me to let go of self-criticism and allow the words to come out have been incredibly rewarding. Her pre-Thanksgiving show in November was called "Gratitude", and it seemed pretty clear that if I was gonna read something, that would be the show. My husband, a playwright and author, has participated in her story salon many times. It was my turn.

A Beautiful Future

The sun was going down and the sky was turning gorgeous shades of pink and orange, with streaks of turquoise and folds of clouds, as the California winter sky tends to do. The light was golden and low and I remember thinking how beautiful it was. Time stood still as I held my phone in my hand, staring at it, waiting for it to ring.

I saw that glow around me and felt it shifting toward where I was on that quiet street, as though it were reaching out six blocks up from the beach in my parked car, sending me a message. Although I was terrified, I was very much alive in that moment. I sat there knowing some kind of bad news was coming and that my life was about to change — the radiologist had said she was "concerned".

But I hoped she was wrong. Oh how I wanted her to be wrong.

And then it rang. With my nervous hand, I answered quickly, trying not to press any wrong buttons due to the shakiness of my pounding heart. A woman's voice from my doctor's office asked if I could schedule an appointment.

"Oh no, can I please speak to the doctor?" I asked, clearly understanding there was only one reason to call me in. The voice on the other end calmly and unemotionally repeated, "She would like you to come in." I said I was available that very minute as I was already in my car and could be there in ten.

Before I started the engine, I called my husband at work and, in a strange whisper, barely able to get the words out, I said, "I think I have cancer, I'm going to the doctor's office now." He said he'd meet me there.

I don't remember parking and in the small elevator I was alone and paced liked a caged animal. Every time since, when I've been back in that elevator, I remember how I felt that day and recall the rippled bump in the elevator floor carpet, thinking they needed to fix that. I don't remember arriving or sitting in the waiting area.

My doctor told me something was abnormal in the biopsy result and I asked her what that meant. She said I had a common form of breast cancer and handed me stapled sheets of paper printed in black and white, which I started to scan immediately.

I remember thinking to myself "how the hell am I going to pencil cancer into my schedule, but what came out of my mouth was, "So, does this mean I am going to have a fucked up breast?" It was the strangest, most rude question I'd ever, or have since, asked a doctor. I felt badly for my outburst, as though somehow I was blaming her for the report. She absorbed my rage for which I later apologized, but it was barely necessary. She understood, and I'm grateful for that.

I asked if there was some kind of medication I could have to calm my nerves because I was in a state of total panic, and dying of a heart attack in her office would probably defeat the purpose of considering cancer treatment. She agreed and prescribed Xanax. Whatever else was said is a blur. My husband texted his arrival as I was leaving, though I have no memory of walking those steps out of there.

I reached the outdoors where my husband was waiting. We said almost nothing, hugged and held each other in a loose kind of way, maybe needing air around how heavy the world suddenly felt. I know he was terrified, and I was saddened that this was his lot in life; his little wife, who had given birth to his two wonderful children, was in a dire situation, and neither of us knew what came next.

We traveled separately to the pharmacy and parked next to each other. He went in to have the prescription filled, and I sat in my car with the driver's side door open a few inches, catching my breath. The sun had set completely and there was darkness all around, except for the parking lot lights.

Surrounded by the quiet blanket of a deep navy sky, I decided to call my parental units. I'm not sure who I called first. It might have been my mother. She immediately cried, her shaky voice telling me she loved me. I remember talking to my dad, who made me repeat maybe two times, exactly what the diagnosis was, as I carefully, and slightly annoyed and exhausted, said "I n v a s i v e d u c t a l c a r c i n o m a", knowing he was going to Google it immediately in the comfort of his home office in New Jersey.

In the days ahead, I gradually told close family, except our kids. Until we had a plan, I wanted to wait to explain it to them. As I told people, I started off by apologizing for having to deliver really bad news.

It was only a few days before Christmas, and we had planned to take a trip to Santa Barbara to visit my mother-in-law. My husband told her over the phone and we had a nice overnight visit, all the while the kids not knowing how tightly wound I was. In those couple of days, I held on and tried with all my might to enjoy being alive. I remember thinking I just wanted this disgusting thing out of my body.

Two nights before we were to leave for Santa Barbara, I was in bed crying into my husband's chest in a way I had never cried before. I was heaving, face soaked from salty tears, embarrassed, terrified, lost in the unknown of my diagnosis. Buried in my husband's long arms that wrap around me like a bear hug, if a bear were gentle and unintimidating, we heard a noise.

I heard stomping and we both looked at each other in the darkness, and sucked in our breath to listen closely — and it happened again. There was thumping in the distance. Chuck got up first and then I followed him down the hall. Our son had thrown up in the living room, barely missing the sofa, splattered vomit on the wood floor and a little bit on the Persian rug. He hadn't even cried out — just fell heavily onto his feet as the force of his body lunged with a powerful outward trajectory. He was instantaneously pale and wiped out. We circled around our son as parents do when a child is sick, and cleaned him up. Chuck told me to go back to bed, and he took care of whatever else happened.

The next day our son rested in the living room and I fed him ice chips after calling the doctor, who informed us that a twenty-four-hour virus was going around. We were determined not to cancel our two-hour drive, so the next night, with the hubby at the wheel, we placed our wobbly sixteen-year-old in the front with the passenger seat tilted back, and in the back seat, his grossed out fourteen-year-old sister, and me, totally discombobulated but hanging on. Still, it seemed better than sitting around waiting for a different reality.

After Santa Barbara, said hubby was on the phone with a relative who had gone through breast cancer about five years before, and our son overheard the conversation as he was saying, "Alicia was just diagnosed...." I was walking down the hall when I saw my shirtless teenager standing with the bathroom door open, holding a brush, staring at the air, with vague tears in his eyes, as he was clearly hearing something unbelievable.

I put my hands on each side of my son's soft arms, walked him gently from the bathroom to my bedroom, and sat him down on the edge of the bed. I looked into his watery eyes and told him that the only reason he didn't know sooner was that we were still planning our next steps. I told him I was being cared for by some of the best doctors in the country (a true fact), he knows how strong I am, and I would — we would — get through this.

I don't remember what he said. That moment will probably always be emblazoned in his mind, or maybe not. Sometimes the brain is good at blocking out terrible moments. Then it was time to tell our daughter. She was calm, and asked, "Is your hair going to fall out?" I answered that it might, and if so, it would grow back.

That's how it all began, alongside life's other random surprises.

Getting a diagnosis around holiday time is a bitch. Messages are taken, but calls take longer to return. Questions linger. Action halts. Finally, as January rolled around, with the help of my awesome doctors, I began the anticipated next steps that would lead me toward an entirely new self, although I didn't know that's what was happening at the time.

I thought I was just getting rid of breast cancer. But last year proved to be much more.

Although I never want to do that again, my perspective broadened in ways I'm not sure I'd ever have slammed into otherwise. I couldn't imagine how I would get through it and often wondered if I would die trying, or if I lived, I'd flip out and become an insane little woman huddling in the corner with my poodle. But after the darkness came crystal clear, sparkling beauty. Each day forward is a miracle, a gift, a new page. It started with that sunset I guess.

(The Dear Dyson letter was added here – a little comic relief never hurts.)

Mostly, what I recall now are the words of encouragement that came my way and got me through the shittiest of times. The first trip my dad took to see me some time around chemo number two of six, he brought me a beautiful small maple wood box with a hinged top, lined in dark velvet.

Inscribed on the box, it says (author unknown):

The most beautiful stones
have been washed by the waters
and polished to brilliance
by life's strongest storms.

The box is shallow inside and I wasn't sure what I'd put in it, but wanted to make it useful. It still holds the narrow strips of double stick wig tape and a fortune cookie message that reads:

Determination is what you need now.

Posted on my office wall is one of my horoscopes from that time which says:

Imagine yourself in a beautiful future,
and keep fleshing out the vision with sparkling details.

So that's what I did. Every so often I remember how lucky I was, and how I had something treatable. It felt like a bad hand to have been dealt, but as the months passed, there was only one way to be: grateful. It's a helluva way to get there, but using up my energy in any other way just doesn't make sense. Pushing

through those blurry, awkward days of chemo I wrote a little
something; a message to myself:

> I am but one small creature on this earth
> I am part of the landscape of flowers
> Each one contributing to the beauty of the whole field of flowers
> unique but swaying in the breeze together
>
> Each one a life force.
> Each flower lives and dies
> and can be appreciated
>
> I am a flower on a hill, with cruel wind blowing me from side
>   to side
> I will weather the storm
> I will grow stronger next season
>
> ...and wouldn't you know it, I did.

I did a little curtsey at the end and the audience clapped. Due to
the bright lights on stage I was unable to see the audience, so I
pretended and looked up every so often as I read. I did see
Chuck's face out there because I knew where he was sitting. I had
not told him what I was going to read. Surprises can be fun.

Reality

Above all, be the heroine of your life, not the victim.
Nora Ephron – Wellesley College Commencement Speech

Internal Organs

Last night I started to feel a sharp pain in my upper left side and it sporadically radiated out to my shoulder. It got me nervous but I figured it might even be, um, gas, because I had eaten breaded fish from Traders Joes that may have caused a little stomach upset. (Yes, I'm back to a healthy embarrassment about bodily functions.)

I woke up this morning and still felt this pain. These things get me very nervous. My oncologist had said that sometimes the way they discover something has spread (aside from routine MRIs and mammograms) is when a patient reports a vague pain that they investigate. She said it usually turns out to be nothing, but that the patient's awareness is often the first step. I press down on this little spot under my ribs on the left and wonder "what organ is that?", so I looked it up. I printed a simple diagram of the human anatomy so I'll know what's what. It seems it is indeed my stomach – surprisingly high up. The liver is on the other side. I am glad for this because somewhere along the way I had heard that if "something" spreads it often shows up in the liver or lungs.

According to The National Cancer Institute Fact Sheet, if breast cancer spreads, it typically goes to bone, brain, liver, and lung. I can't think about this because these thoughts paralyze me, but I want to be informed. I took Mylanta figuring if that makes it go away completely, I'm good.

I must pay close attention to my body. The smallest, strangest sensations are important and can be addressed, as long as I don't deny what I feel. Obviously, regular check-ups (nerve-wracking as they are) are mandatory. I always felt I was aware of my body but then those two little lumps appeared without me having a clue. Awareness is the first step. Maybe fear is still useful. It causes me to pay closer attention.

It's Hard to Admit

I don't like admitting this. I don't wish it on anybody. It was a lousy thing to go through. But cancer gave me a tool. It allowed me to stop holding back, because I had no choice.

As much as my body has been saved, so has my spirit. I even got a tummy tuck and a new hairstyle out of the deal. If I could rewind, I would rather not have had cancer.

But cancer pushed me forward. Cancer gave me permission to immerse in self-love. Cancer gave me permission to be selfish. It's okay to admit it. Even if you had the good fortune of a strong, nurturing upbringing, cancer rearranges your tools.

Because of cancer I learned to reach out for help.

Cancer made me step to the front of the line. It's kind of refreshing. I'm still "me" of course, but with the dial turned up, and the sky has not fallen yet. Although I've had my fill of terror with this whole experience and hope I can enjoy good years ahead, maybe I am a better person for having learned what cancer had to teach.

I am feeling the end of this story. Not *my* end, but the end of how it goes mostly. With six chemotherapy treatments and a surgery or two, there is a path. There are many variations of course, some with more surgeries, some with no surgery, or some with no chemotherapy, and a multitude of variables. For some, breast cancer results in the removal of both breasts, the uterus, ovaries and lymph nodes, which has the potential to set off a spiral of consequences such as chronic lymphedema, hormonal mood swings, not to mention effects from medications typically prescribed for at least five years after the diagnosis. It is amazing what the body can tolerate.

I lucked out not needing radiation. I even had no-radiation-required guilt because it was hard watching my dear friends go through it. But they did, and they're doing great.

I'm looking forward to the Avon Walk in early September. It's a perfect place to walk into the next steps of my life. It's a beautiful place to say goodbye to a rough road.

There is not a day that goes by that I am not reminded in some way of all I've been through. But I live in the moment as much as possible and treat myself with kindness.

The rest is as unknown as what dreams I will have tonight. The rest is *as good as I can let it be*.

I accept the new "me" and all of my imperfections.

Not everyone I meet knows what I've been through. It's my secret. My secret well of knowledge, crazy stuff included.

We Are in the Future

Just saw in the news the other day a device called the "Margin Probe" (looks as phallic as it sounds!) now in use to detect whether surgical margins are clear (no evidence of cancerous cells) during surgery. This is a major breakthrough. Had my surgeon been able to use this device last year during my lumpectomy I might not have needed the mastectomy, although I'm glad to be rid of the troublemaker just the same.

It is wonderful to know that future surgeries might not result in the waiting game for the pathology report which causes intense anxiety, and would avoid additional surgery in order to get a clear margin.

Some Days

I was one of the greeters standing at the doorway taking tickets at Rosh Hashanah temple services tonight. Sometimes, like today, I feel anxious. I feel a need to prove that I'm totally healed now. But sometimes I don't feel that way. Even though we wish for a good new year, L'Shanah Tova, going through the motions of greeting people with a smile weighs down on me somehow. Feeling the glances of knowing eyes, those who are aware of what happened, puts me back in that place of fear and heart-break for all that this body of mine experienced. I'm trying to be alright in the sadness. That I don't have to prove a thing. That I'm fine the way I am. Right now.

It was delightful seeing everyone. People asked how I was feeling and although I remember all that has happened, "Great" was my reply and this time it was true.

The Best Weekend Ever at the Avon Walk

We walked and walked for thirty-three miles through neighbor-hoods, along the beach, and up and down hills in beautiful Santa Barbara. It was an exhilarating, physically challenging experience. The two days were filled with celebration and deter-mination. One of my favorite signs on the back of a truck along the route read *"Big or small, save them all"*, with the Rocky movie theme song "Gonna Fly Now" playing in the background. It was awesome!

The event collectively raised over 4.4 million dollars that will be dispersed throughout Southern California for research and services for women and men who cannot afford them.

There are many organizations to choose from. I'm not a proponent of one over the other, but the length of the walk, location, and tools to fundraise with templates for letters and emails was extremely helpful. There are many causes out there.

If you're lucky enough to survive (anything), pick one, and take action.

The walk had other positive outcomes. My husband and I began walking regularly leading up to the event, and we continue the tradition. My kids cheered me on that weekend and it was wonderful for them to see people taking an active role. It helped our family understand the plight of others and the stories we all have to tell.

Not Too Much

"Not too much" he said when I announced while looking in the mirror on the back of our bedroom door that I was planning on getting a haircut the next day. He was facing his computer involved with fixing some photographs.

I've gotten lots of compliments on my new hair. And that makes me happy because I lost all of it in a matter of two weeks. It was quite a shock to the system. Of course I knew it would fall out because I had started the six rounds of chemo.

But I'm alive and as long as I know I'm angry, or happy, or sad, or frustrated, or whatever else, I know I'm still living.

I'm still shocked sometimes at the depth of my emotions after all this time. It's been almost two years since it all started. That's plenty of time to get on with life and stop whining, right?

My new hairstyle and I have been getting along just fine. But if I think long enough about all of this or come across a pre-cancer photo, I begin to miss my previous hair terribly. It is like a friend who moved away to a foreign country and is never coming back. Not only did my dear friend move away, a complete stranger came to take her place. My new hair is an imposter. It is wavy in some parts, scraggly in others and seems to grow slowly. My hair before was silky straight smooth but limp and I was always irritated at how much effort it took to make it look bouncy. I miss it all the same.

I received compliments on my old hair too. Not long before I was diagnosed I was standing in line at the grocery store at the counter where they sell wonderful prepared foods like stuffed cabbage, lemon chicken, spinach, turkey meatloaf and salmon in a caper and lemon butter sauce, and a man about my age standing next to me in line whispered in my ear that I had beautiful hair. I thanked him politely, even though he may have been flirting with me regardless of the fact that I was wearing a wedding ring. He looked like a decent enough person though, and I carried that compliment around with me for at least a solid week. Little did I know while standing at the counter that day that my hair would soon be gone.

So, I'm standing in front of the mirror that is on the back of our bedroom door realizing that my short hair was becoming unruly. It sneaks up on me the way leg hair tends to do in the winter. If you don't pay close attention after days of wearing jeans and boots, suddenly you realize you've got to take care of things. Looking in the mirror I said I only needed a slight trim on top, just to neaten things up, as it continues to grow into some other style.

"Not too much" my husband said. But what he really meant was, *I want you the way you were before*. He meant that my new boyish style didn't suit him at all.

"Not too much" he said. *Don't get rid of the one thing that helps you look more feminine*, he might have been suggesting.

"Not too much", because if I cut my hair too short it might remind him all over again that I had breast cancer in the first place, and we're trying to make progress here, trying to get back to our regular lives.

"Not too much". *Don't take away any more of you that I love*, he meant. Yes, *that* is what he meant.

Just don't get me started on wishing my eyebrows would grow back.

Last Entry, Otherwise I'll Never Finish This Story
(because it's not really over)

Today is the one-year anniversary of my mastectomy and recon-struction. I'm alright with it. I never expected perfection and it is not. I knew the replacement would never equal what nature came up with. But my new breast is a work of art. The shape and feel are incredibly close to the real thing. The areola tattoo is almost a perfect match to her friend on the right. It was a lot to go through for one small breast. More importantly, I'm alive right now this very minute.

Last night Chuck and I were talking about how my new breast is great and even though it was difficult getting used to I'm so happy and what a difference a year makes. It's incredible.

To which he replied, "Yes it's good but I feel like I'm cheating on you when I touch it". I thought that was hilarious. After all he and I have been through, the least I could do was let him have the (almost) last line in this book, and it's a good place to end this story.

That was one hell of a blip, indeed.

Epilogue

I've never thought of myself as a nervous ninny, fearful that something terrible might happen. But working on the book leaves me with such sorrow. It reminds me of my reality while I am trying to forget. After all this time, I am still afraid.

While doing a little bit of research I am forced to recognize the possibility that cancer can come back. The only way to function is to forget somehow, because to think otherwise sets off a sadness, a lethargy, an ache so deep, I cannot face it. And what saddens me even more is that I don't know if I'd have enough in me to do it again. That maybe if I had a second diagnosis I would then let go. I've met people who have survived more than once. But survival means many things. Some woman are living with stage IV cancer and live treatment to treatment, or test to test. Although I find it to be a desperate situation, the leaps and bounds of modern science gives me great hope despite my worry.

Thankfully I've been told my prognosis is excellent. And by that I mean, my doctors continuously reassured me when I began treatment that I could plan on being an old lady some day. I envision "old" me, with soft gray hair and pink lipstick, holding my poodle, content with the world. But I cannot deny the impact cancer had on my life.

When I was first diagnosed during the winter months I spent a lot of time indoors healing. By late spring I was ready to enjoy the outdoors a little bit and I would sit in our small front garden under the sunshine, acutely aware of how much I had missed of the world around me. I also noticed, almost for the first time, the noise of the cars just feet away from my little spot of earth and the exhaust fumes when someone would pull away from the spot in front of my house. At the height of my paranoia during cancer treatment, I became fearful of my little front garden and sat there less and less. Another year rolled around, and another winter and I stopped thinking of the garden for a while and temporarily forgot about my new anxiety and thoughts of those cars ruining my tranquility.

Now, two years later, I continue to be aware of the cars on my street as they come and go. I am more aware of my surroundings than ever before and have a heightened sense of the dangers lurking in everyday life. I also notice the butterflies and the bees doing their handiwork for another season and wonder what kind of planet we are leaving for our children.

I'll never know if my breast cancer was caused by my state of mind and a failing of my immune system or environmental toxins, or all of the above. I remember the geneticist had said *"Most cancer is caused by environmental factors plus age"* when I questioned how this could have possibly happened to me, a supposedly healthy, BRCA negative, vibrant, young-ish woman.

Although I can't walk around terrified, I feel a sense of urgency, knowing that various types of cancer are associated with our environment. It's a miracle I get through the day. And then I consider the potential hazards we all face and find the resolve to keep going.

Walking along the beach a few blocks from where we live, my husband and I consider ourselves fortunate to be so close to the shimmering ocean. I also go toward a busy intersection now and then so I can pick up a few things and get a workout at the same time. When I cross those streets these days, I tend to cover my mouth and nose with my hand or my sweatshirt sleeve to avoid breathing in the dirty air as a car or bus passes. Even if it doesn't keep out the dust and dirt, it makes me feel better. When my husband sees me do this I tell him, "I might look a little strange but I don't care". So far he hasn't decided to switch to the other side of the street to avoid my slightly weird behavior. I've even considered wearing a mask like people in China, but I don't want to act like a crazy person. And then I think about how awful it must be to really need to wear such masks and that we are all on the same planet together. As I walk back up the hill and watch the line of cars headed toward the nearest freeway, it saddens me that cities all over the world have become so accustomed to polluted air. Underground parking garages are also a source of ridiculous amounts of anxiety for me now, as are the multitudes of other possible toxic chemicals and substances many of us encounter every single day. I've recently joined an organization called Breast Cancer Action which focuses on how products you and I use are regulated. I am optimistic that my involvement will lead to something good, and at the very least, I'll keep learning.

I've also been thinking about what I buy at the supermarket which is at least more in the realm of my control. As author Michael Pollan points out in his book *In Defense of Food*, "*Avoid food products containing ingredients that are unfamiliar, unpronounceable, more than five in number or include high-fructose corn syrup.*"

I had read the book many years before my diagnosis and considered myself to be a healthy eater. My daughter used to ask me if I ate anything besides salad. But there is always room for improvement. I read labels and make the best choices possible while living on the same planet as everyone else. Thankfully the dark chocolate gods shine upon me since it is considered an antioxidant. Hooray for small blessings.

The great news is that my recent meeting with my oncologist was uneventful, just the way we like it. There is a special place in my heart for the nurses and doctors who were so wonderful. Lingering effects from treatment are ringing in my ears (tinnitus) which began around my second chemo and never went away, those damned hot flashes and insomnia thanks to Tamoxifen, body aches for no damned reason whatsoever, intermittent foggy thinking, as well as loss of appetite associated with mild queasiness, and last but not least, bouts of sadness. One of the strangest reminders of all, are my eyebrows. Reduced to a bare thread from hormonal changes and hair loss, there is little pigment left from their once upon a time dark brown, and I now recreate them every morning using pencil and powder. It's a very small price to pay but without drawing them on each day, my face looks similar to the way it did when I lost all of my hair. And then I remember. And my heart sinks a little.

But I can't walk around worrying every minute of every day. That won't do me any good. Being present in the moment is the best way I know to not get bogged down by the *what ifs*.

As long as I can embrace life with authenticity, I believe the rest will fall into place.

Now if you'll excuse me, I'm going to do some cartwheels.

In the grass.

Barefoot.

With the sun on my shoulders.

But not too much. I don't want to get skin cancer.

... almost everything – all external expectations, all pride, all fear of embarrassment or failure – these things just fall away in the face of death, leaving only what is truly important. Remembering that you are going to die is the best way I know to avoid the trap of thinking you have something to lose. You are already naked. There is no reason not to follow your heart.

Apple Co-Founder, Steve Jobs

The Jungle

The cancer jungle keeps you hidden for a while
covered in debris, tall trees blocking the sunshine
But you keep walking
keep on the path
and soon you discover
you have been looking ahead at flowers blooming

Along the way you huddled at night
afraid of unfamiliar sights and sounds
depleted, and you begged the earth and sky
to get you through the brush, the thorns, and the thunder

The sky cried with you in loud claps of rain
and you kept on going
You pushed through mud and rocks and steep hills
You climbed up, over and through to safety
You found nourishment in hidden valleys, you endured it all.
You kept on going each day
And the next

Finally, the sky is getting clearer with each step
You are not covered in darkness
You can see the jungle behind you
You feel the scrapes from the mangled branches
But now, you have found a new path

You have been the warrior of the jungle
You have climbed the mighty hillside
You have found your way

Drink from the stream ahead; the cool, clear water of strength
Bask in the life you have claimed
It was hard work climbing out of the jungle, but you have.

Feel the breeze up ahead
Smell the fragrance of life you hold in your hands
the flowers you have picked
You have done it

You did become the warrior and you stand proud
living with grace, despite the obstacles
You have done it.

Dear Chemotherapy,

Well, it's been about two years since we last saw each other. Of course you know how much I hated you. Of course you know most people think you're an asshole.

But that is not the reason for this letter. I wish to thank you for all of your help. Without you, I would have perished. I appreciate all that you had to do. It must not be fun, being you. You worked me hard and I was terrified when we first met. And look at us now. I'm running free. And I'm sure you're being kept very busy.

I hope one day your position will be eliminated. It seems that in the future, cells will be closely targeted. It wasn't a pleasure to know you, it's true. But what you did for me I'll never forget. My old cells are gone and new ones have taken their place. Thanks for working so hard to get the job done. I tried my best to be cooperative.

I think this is an official goodbye. I hope to never see you again. Chemo dear, you really ought to learn some manners.

Here's to knocking 'em dead (those misbehaving cells that is).

With ambivalence and cheer,

Alicia

The Details

Diagnosed with invasive ductal carcinoma December, 2011 – initially thought to be stage I but actually was stage II. Two tumors each under 2 cm. ER+, PR+, Her2+

Chemotherapy – TCH – Taxotere, Carboplatin, Herceptin

Began Chemo February 15th

Ended Chemo May 30th

Lumpectomy – left side – July 13th

Margins not good enough

Mastectomy – left side – with Flap Reconstruction September 20th

Herceptin – total of 17 sessions

February 12th – Port removed, new nipple, abdominal incision corrected

Tamoxifen for five years – began November 5th

Soul Rocks is a fresh list that takes the search for soul and spirit mainstream. Chick-lit, young adult, cult, fashionable fiction & non-fiction with a fierce twist

Resources

American Cancer Society: www.Cancer.org
Education and Advocacy: www.BreastCancerAction.org
Giving and Receiving Help: www.Lotsahelpinghands.com
Gorgeousness: www.Beautybus.org
Hats, Scarves, Wigs: www.Headcovers.com
Human Hair Wigs: www.Createdhair.com
Navigating Cancer Website: Breast Cancer Blogs:
    www.Navigatingcancer.com/explore/breast/blogs
Well-Being, Nutrition: www.Simmsmanncenter.ucla.edu